# Mind Potential

## *Unzip the Fat Suit Using Your Mind*

*How to change your body permanently,
by easily changing your mind*

## By Maggie Wilde

*Featuring guest fitness experts Sharny & Julius Kieser*

Published by Mind Design Centre Pty Ltd.

© Mind Design Centre & Maggie Wilde 2013

Cover design, book formatting & Ebook conversion by Verbii.com

ISBN: 9780987468307 (Paperback / Softcover)
ISBN: 9780987468321 (E-book)
ISBN: 9780987468338 (Digitised book)

Copies are available at special rates for bulk orders.

Contact info@thepotentialist.com or www.maggiewilde.com

## This book is dedicated to those of us who have ever:

Yo-yo dieted

Used food as comfort

Searched the pantry or fridge when feeling hurt, angry, bored or lonely

Wasted gym memberships or hired exercise equipment that gathered dust

Put alarms on snooze instead of going for a walk

Felt ashamed or embarrassed about their body

Set a goal to lose weight but sabotaged the goal by lunchtime

Regularly wished they hadn't eaten so much

Obsessed about food or weight

Had to finish everything on the plate, even if already full

Wished the latest fad-diet would be the magic pill

Doubted they could ever permanently achieve their goal size, weight and shape

## Once you know how, you *can* get off this merry-go-round and unzip the fat suit permanently

### My thanks go out to:

My incredible clients thank you for trusting me to help.

To the inspirational Trish, you are living proof that all things change. Thank you for helping me help others. Your commitment to your body and health is wonderful, your administration support is priceless, your dedication is breathtaking and your friendship makes my heart sing. To Rachael Bermingham, thank you for your publishing expertise, enthusiasm and mentorship.

To my incredible partner Michael, thank you for your patience and support.

# CONTENTS

Author's Note ........................................................................................ 1

Introduction ......................................................................................... 4

CPR Mind Potential Kit™ ................................................................... 16

Free Audios and Tools

*What is it and how does it work?*

*The CPR Kit includes everything you'll need to Unzip the Fat Suit using your Mind and to create the slim and healthy you permanently.*

*(You can download the CPR Mind potential Kit™ FREE from the link provided. If you would prefer a CPR Mind Potential Kit DVD, it can be ordered from that link also. At various stages throughout the book you will be guided to use the CPR Mind Potential audios, videos and tools appropriately).*

| | | |
|---|---|---|
| **Chapter 1** | The 5 Keys to Think Slim & Healthy - It's all in your mind | 27 |
| **Chapter 2** | Program the Ten Commitments – The Plan! | 47 |
| **Chapter 3** | Control & Conquer Greedy Appetite | 72 |
| **Chapter 4** | Control & Conquer Cravings | 89 |
| **Chapter 5** | Control & Conquer Unhelpful Thoughts, Emotions & Habits | 105 |
| **Chapter 6** | Stop Eating Your Emotions – How to Disconnect Emotions & Food | 126 |
| **Chapter 7** | Rewire Your Inner Image - I'm Gorgeous/You're Gorgeous | 142 |

# Contents

**Chapter 8**    Rewire Digestion - Choose How to Chew ............................ 161

**Chapter 9**    Program – Motivation to Move your Body More .................. 169

**Chapter 10**   Program your Metabolism ..................................................... 185

**Chapter 11**   Program - Once you've zipped it
off you can keep it off ............................................................ 190

**Chapter 12**   Feed the Soul - Unzip Stress and Rewire Calm ..................... 198

**Chapter 13**   Feed the Body - 12 Steps to Healthy
Eating & Perfect Athleticism ................................................. 205

**Chapter 14**   Feed the Mind - Progress Journal to Success ........................ 217


**Appendix** ............................................................................................... 260

**CPR – Mind Potential Kit™ Downloads** ....................................... 261

**Bibliography and recommended reading** ...................................... 262

**About the author and guests** .......................................................... 264

# Author's Note

**Prepare to create 'permanent weight loss' from a unique healthy mind *and* body perspective. Throughout this book, I will show you how to use specific mind strategies in very specific ways. Once you learn these strategies you will be able to unzip the fat suit and take charge of unhelpful eating habits for good. By following this simple plan, those extra kilos will drop away easily, and you will finally create your ideal weight, shape and size permanently.**

**You will achieve that ideal size without dieting, counting calories or measuring food. In fact, this program is not like any other approach you will have ever tried. You are about to learn how to *feed your mind* in a fun and enjoyable way in order to unzip the fat suit and create a slim and healthy mind and body.**

This means that while you're using the strategies and solutions in the book, you are also learning what it means to *accept, and even love your body,* as it becomes slimmer and healthier. The free audios provided help you use your mind to think and behave in slim and healthy ways naturally. You are about to learn how to feed your mind back to health, to manage old eating patterns that challenge you and free yourself to think, behave and feel like a slim and healthy person. So be patient with your body and mind as you learn how to approach the 'weight loss' experience from a whole new healthy and joyous perspective.

This book will help you shift your perspective and focus from *'having to* or *needing* to *lose weight'*, to '**wanting to** and easily *gaining health'*.

- What if this excess 'fat suit' was just a suit you've been wearing like a costume?
- What if you could learn how to take that 'costume' off and leave it off?
- What if the 'real you' was meant to be slimmer and healthier?
- What if you've gained the extra kilos, lost them, and gained them back again in the past, because you didn't know the simple strategies to unzip them for good?

**You can unzip the excess weight permanently. You can become slim and healthy on the inside,** *from your mind,* **while your physical body catches up to your mind's new healthy slim perspective.**

It's time to become a better friend to yourself while you learn how to help your body be what you want it to be.

◆

Dear reader

I am not perfect; I am as flawed as the next person. However, what I do know is this: once I am aware that something is holding me back from what I want, I have the strategies, technology and solutions to let that flaw go. I have learned how to *control, program and rewire* my mind in very helpful ways.

I'll explain in detail what I mean by **control, program and rewire (CPR)** very soon. Using this CPR strategy is an important key to creating the permanent body, weight and shape that you want.

Over the years I have put my mind, body and spirit through a hell of a journey to get to this point. I initially developed every strategy and solution in this book to help me.

I too had to learn how to be a better friend to my body and unzip the layers I had built around myself. Those layers consisted of extra kilos on my body, weighed down by added physical and emotional pain, resentment and anger, topped off by extremely unhelpful eating habits. These layers all led to a super 'bonus' layer of self-doubt in my mind. If I was to ever finally achieve what I wanted, I needed to choose something different for myself. I had to find ways to use the untapped power of my mind and become kinder to my body and myself too.  When I did this, I gained health in more ways than one.

By reading and using the strategies in this book and the free *CPR Mind Potential audios,* you will not only gain insight into some of my own experiences, but those of clients that I have worked with too. I was physically overweight into my teens and twenties, but I was mentally and emotionally overweight for much longer.

Like many of my clients, I struggled with yo-yo dieting and I was embarrassed about my body too. After years of depression, ill health and resentment, my body eventually became burdened with disease. My eating habits were poor and my self-doubt and fears were many. My body was weighed down with that protective costume I called the 'fat suit'.

As I learned the strategies and developed the tools to unzip that costume, I discovered a healthier attitude towards myself and I learned to appreciate my body. My body seemed to appreciate me more too. I became slimmer and healthier, and I've been working with thousands of clients ever since to do the same with them.

And so it began…

Remember, I am not perfect; I still need to work on my own issues every day in order that I can continually be a better version of myself. However what I know now, is that once I recognise I have a flaw and I work out how it's affecting me; I have the strategies, the technology and the solutions to help me overcome it. My hope, is that at least some of these solutions will find their way to you through this book to help you create a healthy heart, mind and body too.

This is your chance to learn how to use the potential of your mind to unzip the fat suit for good and take control of your eating patterns. This is your chance to find the slim and healthy you permanently! Enjoy discovering the real you!

# Introduction

You are about to discover how to permanently feed your mind and body for healthier habits and outcomes that you've always wanted. You will discover how to build motivation, respect and self-belief to create the health and body you have always desired. Most importantly, by the end of this book, you will know how to keep it that way!

---

*"In order to change the body permanently we must also discover how to change the mind." Maggie Wilde*

---

**Important Note:**

- Before you begin the journey into this book please note that it ***does not*** provide a d...i...e...t...for you to follow
- This book *does not* ask you to beat yourself up about whether you do the d...i...e...t thing right or wrong *(you might tell from this that I intensely dislike diets)*
- This book *does not* ask you to count calories
- This book *does not* ask you to measure food
- This book *does not* ask you to deny yourself anything
- This book *does not* ask you to starve your body
- This book *does not* ask you to only drink cabbage water on Tuesdays and the juice of three grapefruits with a twist of lemon and the rind of a lime on Friday...

If that is really what you want, you've got the wrong book.

This book, is the key to understanding and putting into action how to unzip the fat suit for the last time. It is the key to understanding how to use your mind to support you, rather than work against you. It will help clarify why the world is filled with yo-yo dieters, and why every diet or weight loss program you or your friends have ever tried, may have started well at first and then fallen away in the end. It is the key to understanding why diets don't work. It is the key to why we lose motivation and focus no matter how determined we were yesterday; why we can make a promise to ourselves to exercise one day, and why we stay in bed with the alarm on snooze the next. It is the key to understanding how to change what doesn't work, and reinforce what does.

Your mind holds the blueprint of every cell of your body, what it looks like, how it feels and what it is capable of. The part of you, which is your mind - the thinker, the analyser, the feeler, the doer and the observer - starts being programmed from before you were born. It is programmed with attitudes, perceptions and beliefs that determine your behaviours, your reactions, your emotional intelligence and your ability to deal with life's challenges effectively. Even the method you use to respond to challenges such as whether you turn to comfort food, or react with anger or sabotage, is programmed.

Your brain holds within it patterns, networks of electrical currents called neural pathways that are programmed to stimulate specific thoughts, feelings, actions and reactions to the world around you. These patterns determine your perceptions and beliefs about what you can and can't achieve, what your body does or does not look like, how you do or do not react to that and, how you will or will not live out your life.

## Your Brain's Map

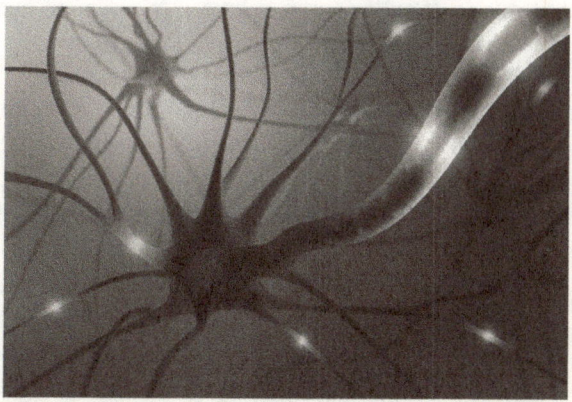

I call this network of patterns in the brain 'your map'. Your map is the blueprint that determines why you stay in bed when your body really needs to move. It rules why you choose chocolate or unhealthy carbohydrates, when your body really needs leafy greens. It has the keys to why you procrastinate, feel unmotivated and sabotage or dislike what you see in the mirror, when you really need to love and nurture your body to health.

If the part of you that is the subconscious mind has been programmed or wired early in life with unhelpful maps, and you have developed inappropriate patterns and perceptions about exercise, health, food, emotions or your body, then your brain has developed a deeply engraved blueprint that causes you to continue repeating those unhelpful patterns and behaviours. Often, if you lose weight, that blueprint recreates the over weight size of your body and the attitude you have about it again and again. Hence the unhelpful cycle of yo-yo dieting that many people experience.

If these patterns go unchecked, you will continue to replay unhealthy programs about why you eat, when you eat, what you eat and how much you eat. If unchecked, they will continue to run the blueprint of the fat suit. So no matter how much weight you lose, you can gain and lose it again and again. If these patterns go unchecked they can also determine your unhelpful thoughts or judgements about your body.

If these patterns were set in stone, then we would be helpless to change anything about our life or our body. There would simply be no point in setting goals for improvement. We would continue to be a product of every yes or no that we have ever said in our lives, prior to this day. If our brains were wired in a pattern that has said yes to chocolate every day for the past twenty years, then we would be a product of that blueprint. If our program had been to say no to exercise for the past 20 years, then we would forever be a product of that too.

**The good news is that there are strategies and solutions you can use to *control, re-program and rewire* these patterns and blueprints.**

What determines whether you continue to say yes or no to unhealthy thoughts and actions is within your power to control, reprogram and rewire. Every attitude, habit, emotion or belief that has been unhelpful to your health and the size of your body, can be changed. When you have the strategies and skills to do this, you can control and stop unhealthy thoughts, habits, cravings or emotional states easily. You can rewire your brain and program your mind and body for better eating habits. You can rewrite neural pathways in the brain that will stimulate motivation to exercise. You can activate the ability to *choose* healthy options and smaller portions and even increase your metabolic rate too. Once you know how to rewire the patterns and blueprints, then your thinking, your behaviour and your emotional reactions will refocus on gaining health. You'll wonder why indeed, excess weight was ever an issue in the past.

As you journey through the book, you will understand your mind and how it currently works. You will then be able to recognise any subconscious behaviours, habits, thought patterns, emotions or beliefs that are helping you move towards slim and healthy, and which ones are moving you away from it.

The *CPR – Mind Potential audios* will help you control, program and rewire the things that are not helping you, and of course, reinforce the ones that are.

Everything you need in order to create this lifelong ability to be slim and healthy is contained within this book and the CPR Mind Potential audios.

Each of the later chapters outline various strategies and provide a step-by-step opportunity for you to change your mind and change your body permanently. By the time you complete the book, you will have everything you need. Your focus will automatically shift from the stress of '*having to lose weight*', to the ease of choosing to '*gain health, to be slim and healthy always*'.

## Internal Conflict?

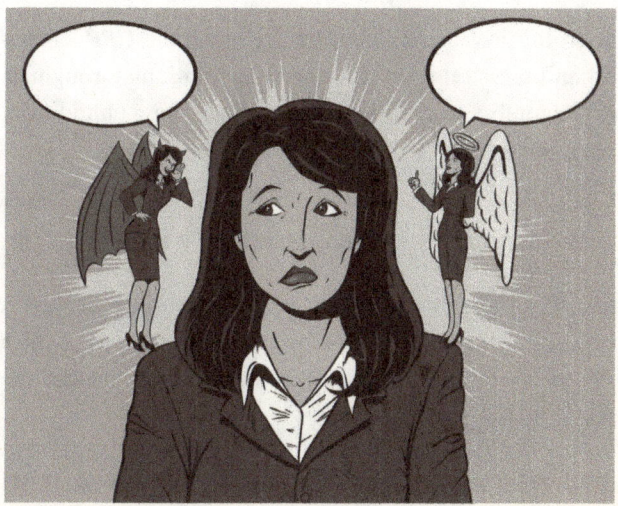

7

As a Mind Potentialist and a specialist in how to modify unhelpful behaviours, attitudes and reactions, I have worked with thousands of clients who deal with inner conflict concerning their body. When this inner conflict occurs, their actions and behaviour can often seem at odds with their desires and goals.

It is as though a part of them would set a goal to reduce weight, however another part created behaviours and thoughts that were at odds with that goal. Part of them would choose to take salad to work for lunch, and that other part would persist in saying yes to the donuts on offer or the snacks at morning tea. Part of them would keep them in bed, when last night they had committed to rise half an hour earlier to exercise. When they felt stressed or upset, that part would continue to reach for comfort food; no matter how determined the healthy part had been to deal with stress differently now. The healthy part that made a New Year's resolution, and the other part that said "oh well, there's always next year".

Although this may sound as if many of us are burdened with dual identities at war with each other, I assure you that the majority of people who have not already achieved what they want, deal with internal conflict too.

In fact, I spent most of the first 35 years of my life in a constant internal battle between the healthy part that wanted life, success, happiness and health versus the confused self-sabotaging part that created self-blame, unhealthy cravings and no motivation to move my body.

## There is good news again:

There is a solution for this internal conflict. By using the *CPR - Mind Potential* audios provided and the strategies and practical solutions throughout the book, you can resolve the conflict and reprogram and rewire for a united front. The little battle in your head will cease.

## The most common mistakes people make when reducing weight

I have provided a list of the most common mistakes people make in order to help you identify them if they appear as you move forward. As part of the book I outline the strategies to overcome these mistakes, so you can be the healthiest version of yourself that it is possible to be.

The processes outlined are designed to help you reframe or delete mistakes before they happen, and successfully conquer every one of them for the future.

## Mistake 1:     Skipping meals

Make sure you eat three small meals everyday. When you skip meals and don't consume enough kilojoules, it causes your body to go into starvation mode. This is not a myth, your metabolism becomes sluggish, and the automatic subconscious processes instruct your body to store fat in order to protect it from starvation.

## Mistake 2:     Setting unrealistic time frames and goals

Be realistic in setting the time frame to reach your goal. Do go for your ultimate weight and shape, aim for your idealistic you, simply do it in a realistic time frame. I have a client who has lost over 70 kilograms. No one, including her, thought she would ever achieve such a goal. She did this by: *setting realistic time frames and smaller chunk goals*. She first set 10 kg goals; she would only focus on that next 10 kg goal.

As she moved closer to her ideal weight, shape and size, she set smaller incremental goals of 5kgs. With the last few kilograms, I asked her to focus only on being under the next kilo, this way her mind could cope with the change without becoming over-whelmed. When she first realised she had 70kgs to lose, she would lose a few kilos and then give up because it all seemed too hard. Once the goals and the timeframe were realistic, her mind cleared and she was able to focus and feel motivated. (At the time of writing this book she has let go of over 77 kg *(half her original body weight)*.

## Mistake 3:     Only focused on short term results, it is important to re-assess your 'Why'

This means *if you use the date of a wedding as the time frame* to unzip the fat suit, then be aware that your goal has an end date. You therefore need to regularly assess your - *'why' do you want to be healthy* - along the way.

If you reach the wedding day and you achieved your goal, but you haven't reas-sessed your 'Why' do I want to *stay healthy*, it can often go backwards. Or if you didn't quite achieve your goal by the wedding date, then your motivation to keep going needs to be attached to a different goal. In order to succeed you need a dif-ferent 'Why' to keep going. It is important to reassess this 'Why' regularly until being slim and healthy becomes so deeply ingrained, that you eventually become the kind of person who *is* slim and healthy permanently. (I'll discuss the impor-tance of your 'Why' in Chapter 1).

## Mistake 4:    Being too busy to stick to the program or exercise

Hmmm for me being 'too busy' to be healthy is simply an excuse. It simply means the *'Why'* I want to be healthy is not powerful enough yet. In order to prioritise being slim and healthy, you need to focus on a powerful emotional connection to the reasons you want to achieve that. You must have a strong emotional connection to your motivating factor. If your motivating factor is powerful enough, then you will begin to prioritise the things you need to do so that you can achieve the outcome.

---

*"If you want it bad enough you will find ways to make it happen, if you don't you will make excuses instead." Anonymous*

---

## Mistake 5:    Weighing too often

Only weigh in once per week. I'll discuss this more as part of YOUR PLAN in the Ten Commitments in Chapter 2.

## Mistake 6:    Going it alone

Research shows when you have support and make yourself accountable, you are more likely to succeed in everything you do. I suggest you work with a buddy who wants to do this too, or email info@thepotentialist.com to discuss other online options to help you.

## Mistake 7:    Calorie intake becomes the focus.

If calorie intake is the primary concern and you disregard the importance of what your mind hears, thinks and sees, then success is often short lived. When your internal body image is not addressed, the results are often limited. Eventually 'famine gives way to feast' and the weight goes back on. This issue is definitely addressed in a variety of ways throughout the book and in the CPR audios.

**Mistake 8:**     **Unhelpful emotional attachments to food and eating are not addressed.**

This book and the CPR audios address emotional attachments as a priority. I include in this, the relationship between food and stress, boredom, comfort, habitual and other unhelpful emotional triggers.

**Mistake 9:**     **Unhelpful beliefs about food and the body are not addressed.**

This too is definitely a focus throughout this book and the CPR audios. Addressing any unhelpful belief systems *(for example: "I'll never get this weight off" or "I won't be able to keep it off")* is vital in order to achieve permanent change.

**Mistake 10:**     **Procrastination and excuses have not been addressed.**

Ditto. Providing practical solutions and strategies to overcome these issues is an important part of this book and the audios.

**Mistake 11:**     **Resistance to exercise and the inability to sustain motivation**

This subject is one of the most discussed topics in my clinics; in fact, resistance to exercise or the ability to sustain the motivation to do it regularly, challenges many people. This is so important that I have provided specific *Program and Rewire* audios designed to motivate you to move your body more. These audios have been designed to help you overcome this resistance once and for all.

**Mistake 12:**     **Dieting becomes the focus**

Research shows that diets don't work. When you *go on* something, you are programmed to know one day you will *come off* it. This spells disaster to me. If you haven't learned how to change the things that didn't work before, you'll keep doing the same things, and therefore repeatedly create the same outcomes.

## Mistake 13:   Fears about putting the weight back on and self-doubt or self-blame are not addressed.

Why do you think the weight loss world has so many quick fix cures? Every client that comes to my clinic has attempted at least five (if not more) different *diets or weight loss* programs. They're coming to me because the diets either didn't work or only worked for a short time. The minute they *went off* the other program, they put the weight (if not more) back on. I address this issue with specific Control audios and further strategies in the book.

## Mistake 14:   Obsession with weighing and measuring food.

For many of us, weighing and measuring food is too restricting to maintain. Once the initial '*why* **do I want to reduce weight**' has been achieved, there is no reason to continue counting, measuring or restricting, so the weight goes back on. Often the original goal is never attained, because the obsession and time consuming preparation becomes tiresome. When we can't be bothered weighing or measuring anymore, the '*I failed*' or '*I'm hopeless*' or '*I'll never get this weight off*' syndrome is reinforced.

## Mistake 15:   Denying /restricting food is seen as the solution.

For many of us, when we deny or say we can't have this or that, we activate that little rebellious monkey in our head that says, *"don't tell me what to do"*. It is important to understand *there are no banned foods, simply less of them and less often*. The CPR audios are designed to help you rewire your automatic instinct to choose healthier options and smaller portions anyway.

## Mistake 16:   The focus is on 'losing weight', instead of 'gaining health'.

When we 'lose' something we are pre-programmed to find it again...d'oh! Also the interpretation of 'lose' can often have negative connotations at the subconscious level. *(Perhaps we lost something in the past that we originally associated with grief, sadness, failure, anger and frustration)*. At the subconscious level, most of us don't really want to *lose*, especially if loss caused feelings of angst or sorrow in the past.

'Lose weight'. Say it silently in your mind now. What does it 'feel' like? Often we are left with a heavy sensation after saying those words. On the other hand, when you say 'gain health' you will feel 'lighter' somehow. Try it out now. *'Gain Health'*. Let's do it!

**My Unzip the Fat Suit Program takes the holistic approach to weight reduction.**

By unzipping the fat suit in your mind, your emotional state, your belief system and your thoughts, actions and habits, you can ensure that all parts of you are working towards the same outcome. The entire system that is you (your mind, body and spirit), will become the *kind of person who is* slim and healthy. A slim and healthy person eats less, they move more and they automatically like what they see in the mirror.

## Having a Plan - The 10 Commitments

As part of the Mind Potential - Unzip the Fat Suit approach, I also provide a chapter dedicated to the importance of having a plan. When working towards slim and healthy, there are 10 very simple Commitments that make up your plan. Those 10 Commitments are the steps you will follow to achieve the outcome you desire.

In Chapter 2, I outline those 10 Commitments and explain the importance of the audios and where they fit into the commitments to support you in your quest for slim and healthy. The CPR audios are specifically designed to reinforce the 10 Commitments. They will help to program the foundation of the commitments and rewire the neural pathways to help you choose to action those commitments easily. You will simply begin to think like a slim and healthy person by following the 10 Commitments and using the CPR audios. How to use the CPR audios, will be outlined in detail immediately following the Introduction.

Once you understand the importance of the 10 Commitments and the vital role of the CPR audios and you begin to use them, the control, program and rewire processes happen automatically.

**Remember: the audios motivate you to choose to do the 10 Commitments and the 10 Commitments motivate you to choose to do the audios. It's a win / win outcome.**

My intention as a therapist in clinic is to help clients achieve their outcome in the healthiest, shortest and most effective way. My intention with this book and the CPR audios, is to help you achieve your outcome in the healthiest, shortest and most effective way too.

In doing this, I also need to address the relationship you currently have with food, eating and your body. The key outcomes I intend for you as the reader include:

- To help you build your confidence, and a deep knowing within, that you can be slim and healthy, and stay that way
- To help you understand the role *you play* in controlling, programming and rewiring your mind and body for slim and healthy actions
- To help you realise and believe how easy it is to achieve your ideal weight, shape and size permanently
- To help you see the importance of your self-image, the importance of how your brain processes what you look like and who you think you are, and how you feel about yourself and your body

It is important to understand the roles that both our conscious (rational thinking part), and subconscious (automatic internal reactions and responses such as hunger, digestion, unconscious habits) play in our health. When we understand the responsibility we have in shaping our body's weight, shape and size, we can begin to recognise the importance of addressing our unhelpful habits and behaviours in ways that we haven't done before.

When we address our responsibility to ourselves in this way, and we understand how to make that a priority, then we are well on the way to achieving what we wish for.

## Wishing and wanting versus actually doing

This book, the 10 Commitments and CPR audios, also help you address the shift from *wishing and wanting to be slim and healthy,* to actually *creating it*. I provide strategies and audio technology to build motivation, self-belief, to change unhelpful habits and conquer unhelpful cravings as you make your way towards health. I address how you can build a better relationship with your body, and how to become a better friend to yourself. How to easily make healthier choices because you choose it to be so, not because you have to, or should do.

I also address your relationship with food and eating, your past beliefs or any perceptions that may no longer be helpful to the healthy outcome that you choose to create. The book addresses doubts, fears and frustrations, stress, judgement and *'will-power or won't-power'*. I help you approach the slimmer, fitter, healthier you from every angle, including appropriate movement of your body, healthier options to put into it, and the motivation to do so.

## In summary

To change your body permanently, you must also learn how to use and change your mind in positive, health directed ways. This book, the Ten Commitments and the CPR audios, will lead you effortlessly through that process. Most importantly, you will learn how to keep it that way!

This book will outline how to understand your mind and how it currently works. The CPR audios, the Ten Commitments and all of the other strategies provided, help you change, program and rewire the unhelpful behaviours, habits, thoughts, emotions and beliefs that are not moving you toward your goal, and reinforce the ones that do.

Welcome to the ride of your life… Maggie Wilde

# CPR Mind Potential Kit™

## What is it, and how does it work?

### *The Good News*

The *CPR Mind Potential Kit™ contains mind potential strategies and a variety of self-hypnosis audios and videos with powerful slim and healthy suggestions. In comparison to using diets or supplements alone, research studies show that when people use hypnosis techniques to support weight loss, their results more than double. By using the Mind Potential CPR audios and strategies, (which contain hypnotherapeutic techniques), you will unzip the fat suit easily and learn how to think slim and healthy for good.*

The CPR Mind Potential Kit™ contains:

1. A selection of **Control, Program and Rewire Mind Potential Audios and Videos**. These are created specifically to help you reprogram your mind to think like a slim and healthy person. To see yourself from the inside as slim and healthy. To feel motivated to move your body, control and eliminate unhelpful cravings or sabotaging habits and choose healthier options. To believe in yourself and your ability to stay slim and healthy for good.
2. Demonstration Videos to Control Cravings and other helpful strategies.
3. Easy strategies you can use to achieve permanent weight reduction using your mind.

Once you understand the importance of the CPR audios and videos, and you begin to use them, new positive habits, behaviours and healthier choices become automatic for you. You begin to think positively, you begin to encourage yourself more with helpful self-talk, supporting yourself to make healthy choices and motivating yourself effortlessly to move your body more.

The CPR Mind Potential Kit™ and the Mind Potential Audios are specifically designed to control and conquer any *unhelpful* neural pathways in your brain (the electrical circuitry), then program and rewire *more helpful* circuitry to achieve better attitudes, habits and beliefs about food and exercise for the rest of your life.

*Please Note: These techniques are not a substitute for medical care or dietary advice and the CPR Mind Potential audios and videos will produce a pleasant relaxed feeling and light trance experience, so they should not be used while driving a car or operating machinery. If you suffer from, or have ever been diagnosed with a chronic medical condition, epilepsy or a psychological disorder, please consult with your medical or mental health care practitioner before using the CPR programs. If in doubt, ask your medical practitioner before you begin if hypnotherapeutic techniques and self-hypnosis are appropriate for your use.*

## CPR – Mind Potential Kit™

## Control – Program – Rewire

The three CPR audio and video technologies and what they each contain are:

## Technology One: Control & Conquer Audios

*Control and Conquer* audios and the other Control strategies in the book are designed to put you back in control of your choices and habits. The Control audios help you stop unhelpful cravings and habits that have kept you from achieving your ideal weight. These audios help you stop the unhelpful emotional eating patterns and thoughts. They help control issues such as:

- Chocolate or sweet cravings
- Starchy carbohydrate urges
- Overeating, snacking, grazing or picking
- Addictions to fast foods, fizzy drinks and takeaways
- The need for cakes, sweets, lollies, ice-cream, biscuits
- Late night grazing or snacking in-between meals
- Unhelpful angers, frustrations, emotional, comfort or stress eating
- Any unhelpful connection between emotions and food

By using the ***control and conquer*** audios and videos, you will interrupt the trigger that caused the craving or addiction, which means that you will be able to break old unhelpful patterns easily. By using the audios and watching the demonstration videos you can instantly stop unhelpful thoughts, emotions, habits and behaviours and feel more in control of what you eat and why you eat it.

Contained within the Mind Potential Kit there are a number of Control audios to listen to and implement. If you prefer learning visually I have provided demonstration videos of these too. By using the control audios and other exercises in the book, you'll be able to say no to unhealthy eating habits with ease.

Keep your eye on my websites: www.thepotentialist.com or www.maggiewilde.com and YouTube channel: *Maggie Wilde*: http://www.youtube.com/MaggieWilde as I often update or add to the free demonstration audios and videos.

## Technology Two: Program Audios

These Audios program your mind to lay the foundation you need to think like a slim and healthy person thinks. They will help you build the confidence and determination you need and they will help you eliminate unhelpful stress. They help to motivate you in order to turn 'will-power' into effortless 'choice-power'.

**By using Program audios you will develop the power to *choose* slim and healthy, because you *want it*, instead of feeling as though you *have* to.**

Program your mind for slim and healthy with a selection of my Program Audios contained in the kit. They include:

- Eliminate Greedy Appetite (Includes reinforcement of the 10 Commitments – refer to Chapter 2)
- Motivation to Move your Body and Exercise
- Be Stress Free

As you repeatedly listen to each of these audios your mind begins to create the healthier you from the inside. The foundations of neural connections are laid in order to help you create the healthier habits, thoughts and beliefs required to be slim and healthy.

## Technology Three: Rewire Audios

Use these audios while you walk, workout or relax. These shorter audios rewire neural pathways (your brain's electrical circuitry) for ***permanent change***. These audios take advantage of some of the ways in which the brain learns including repetition, rhythm, sensation and subliminal beats. By using these you will automatically learn to think and feel like a slim and healthy person thinks and feels.

Rewire your mind easily with these audios provided in the CPR Mind Potential Kit. They include:

- **Rewire for Slim and Healthy - Unzip the fat suit** – I have provided the cardio version of this audio to use while you work out ***and the*** relaxation version to chill out and enjoy. Both versions stimulate your mind to learn everything you need. They include reinforcement of your plan (the 10 Commitments detailed in Chapter 2).
- **Rewire for Confidence – Build Confidence and Self Esteem** – Once again you can use either the relax edition or pump it to the cardio version while you walk or work out. Your mind will love the stimulation while it reprograms and rewires to be slim, healthy and confident permanently.

The CPR - Mind Potential Kit™ containing deep hypnotherapeutic suggestions helps create the slim and healthy you that you have always wanted. Sit back and relax while you let your mind do the work for you. Each of these audios reinforces healthier concepts, they provide the technology you need to remove resistance, and create the healthy motivation you need to keep going.

## How CPR Audio Technology Works

In order to unzip the fat suit permanently it is important to have an understanding of the methods your mind and brain uses to learn. When you understand and implement these methods you will allow your mind to work ***with*** you to achieve that healthy and slim body.

Once you begin to take the appropriate actions towards your ideal goal, whether that goal is to reduce 5 kg or 50 kg, the only way to maintain that outcome is to change your perception of yourself too. To ensure your success is permanent, you must learn how to control, program and rewire your brain to not only *think* like a slim and healthy person, but to *see yourself as slim and healthy,* and to *believe* it too.

Too often I hear stories from clients who had previously lost and gained 10-30 kg perhaps 3 or 4 times. No matter how much they lost they still had a 'fat internal perception' of their body. They still saw and thought of themself as fat. Until this mental impression is changed, the slim and healthy you cannot become permanent. This is why it is vital to reprogram your self-image and self-perception along the way. The solutions in this book and CPR audios help you do this.

Take this opportunity to become the kind of person who *is slim and healthy*, rather than the kind of person who *wishes they were but doubts they can be, or* doubts they will maintain it. Sound familiar?

Your progress will become effortless when you apply the strategies in the book, do the 10 Commitments – YOUR PLAN (Chapter 2) and listen to the audios as and when suggested.

### CPR audios and video demonstrations in summary:

**To ensure all parts of you work toward the one healthy outcome you need all three: CPR - Mind Potential Kit Technologies:**

**C = Control & Conquer Audios** *(Control & Conquer Cravings & Unhelpful Emotional Eating Habits & Thoughts)*

**P = Program Audios** *(Program Your Mind for Slim & Healthy – these audios lay the foundation so that your mind knows exactly how to help you)*

**R = Rewire Audios** *(Rewire for Permanent Change – these audios use the brain's capacity to learn by using repetition, sensation and rhythm to rewire your brain for lasting change)*

Use them as prescribed and you will unzip the fat suit and create the slim and healthy you in no time. Let's find out how...

# How often should I use the CPR audios?

Use at least one audio once per day.

At different stages within the book, there will be certain audios that are relevant to the issues being addressed. I'll outline which ones to use and when to start them.

**Audio one**: Start today with the first Program audio 'Eliminate Greedy Appetite'. This will introduce all the principles needed including smaller portions, healthier options, feeling fuller faster on far less food, chewing more slowly, drinking more water, motivation to move the body more, being in control of what, when, why and how much you eat. It suggests ways to reprogram your ideal weight, shape and size in the control room of your mind. It sets up the process for the rest of the audios to take you deeper into that learning.

Use the 'Eliminate Greedy Appetite' Audio at least once per day for 5 days and then as often as you wish. I suggest at least twice weekly from there, as we begin to add the other audio programs too. There are no 'have to's' here. You decide what feels right for you to use. All the audios help you move towards the ideal you! Mix and match them, use what feels right today or what's needed to address a particular issue.

**Health Bonus:** research shows that using these types of techniques is beneficial for general health and wellbeing. Used regularly they help to lower unhealthy blood pressure and cholesterol; they create a more balanced sense of wellbeing and a positive outlook on life in general. They increase metabolic rate *(bonus for this purpose)*, reduce stress and improve sleep patterns. These are just some of the many benefits of using CPR audios, not to mention becoming the ideal weight, shape and size you wish to be.

**Using CPR Audios Guideline**:

1. Use at least one Program and one Rewire audio every day for 31 days (more often if you have time to do so)
2. *Use Control* audios as and when required helping you manage unhelpful cravings and emotions. (This will be explained in Chapter 3)
3. Use Program audio– *'Eliminate Greedy Appetite'* from day one. Listen once per day for at least 5 days then alternate with other Program audios for at least 31 days
4. Use Program audio - *'Motivation to Move your Body & Exercise'* from day 6. Alternate this with 'Eliminate Greedy Appetite' as often as you choose. If finding motivation to exercise is an issue for you please use this audio until this issue has been addressed appropriately

5. Add to that Rewire audio one and two –*Rewire for Confidence and Rewire for Slim and Healthy.* Use one of these at least once per day alternating them as you wish for the first 31 days then as often as you choose. These Rewire audios are shorter than the program tracks so you may wish to use them more than once per day initially

6. As your body lets go of excess kilos it is very important to de-stress and stay calm because the calmer you are the faster your results will be (refer to Chapter 14). Therefore, I have included a bonus Program audio – *Be Stress Free* to help you manage and reduce stress levels and reduce weight faster.

   a. Add *'Be Stress Free' Program Audio. Alternate this with Program audios one and two as often as you wish.*

*(There are many other optional audios that can be purchased from the website to support your journey if you wish. Titles such as: Liposuction Using The Mind, Emotional Release, Release Anger and Resentment, Let Go Self-Sabotage and more)*

## When is the Best Time to Use the Audios?

The best time to use them is when it suits you. Last thing at night or first thing in the morning is great. But If I tell you to only use the CPR audios before you get up in the morning, but morning is your busiest time of the day, then the likelihood that you will use them regularly, is slim.

Pick a time when it's quiet and you won't be disturbed. Use earphones so that you won't disturb anyone else and sit up comfortably to listen. If you are listening in bed, as the track nears the end, snuggle down and drift off to a natural, deep sleep. The positive thoughts or images of the program will continue to flow through your mind while you sleep.

## Should I listen to them with earphones?

Yes, the most benefit will be gained if you do listen to them with earphones. There are deep subconscious layers of rhythm and a hypnotic heartbeat within the programs, so using earphones will enhance this experience. You can upload the audios to your iPod, iPhone, mp3 player, computer, laptop or other device.

## What if I Fall Asleep When I Use Them?

If this happens every now and then, that is absolutely fine. If you do fall asleep while listening often, then attempt to sit more upright or use the audios at a different time of the day if that's possible. Make an effort to listen to the audios semi-consciously all the way through every now and then.

## How Can I Gain the Most Out of the CPR Audios?

Be open to the suggestions and allow them in. If your analytical conscious mind tries to distract you, simply acknowledge that you are going to listen anyway. Even if you can't believe the suggestions yet, let them in by pretending. If your mind drifts off that's perfect too. Use this as timeout to 'play', pretend and 'act as if' the suggestions are real. Have fun with them and you will feel and see the benefits faster.

## Fake it till you make it

To enhance the effectiveness of the audios it is simply your role to engage in the suggestions '*as if*' they are real. You learn faster and more effectively when you add sensations, feelings and emotions to the experience. Act as if you are a child innocently hearing what you hear, as if it is real, right now.

Even if you can't believe the new slim and healthy ideas and images yet, engage anyway by allowing yourself to experience the journey. Feel what you feel, see what you see, and hear what you hear. The more you allow the suggestions in and engage your senses in the process, the more quickly and effectively the healthy new neural pathways in your brain will be established.

*Your brain learns by engaging positive sensory input (feelings, sensations and emotions), repetition and rhythm, so let yourself engage as much as you can, and the change will happen easily.*

## When Shouldn't I Use the Audios?

Never use the audios while driving a car or using machinery. It is important also to consult with your medical or mental healthcare practitioner before starting the CPR audio programs if you have a psychological issue, epilepsy or a serious health condition. If you are in any doubt about using these audios, please consult your medical healthcare practitioner first.

## How do I get access to the CPR Mind Potential Kit™?

- The following download link will take you to a registration page on my website. Register your name and email address and I will send you your personal password to access the *FREE CPR Mind Potential Kit™*. The kit includes all audios, videos and other amazing tools you will need to be slim and healthy permanently.
- If you would prefer an Unzip the Fat Suit Using Your Mind - CPR Mind Potential DVD, just drop us a line at info@thepotentialist.com or use the same link provided and there will be an option to request a FREE DVD to be posted to you. All you'll pay is $5.00 postage and handling and the DVD kit is yours free.

## CPR Mind Potential Kit Download Link: *http://www.thepotentialist.com/cprkit/*

- You will be guided at different stages throughout the book to use different audios, strategies and solutions from the CPR Mind Potential Kit™. The book will show you how to use the audios and videos step-by-step.

## CPR Mind Potential Kit Content List

## Control Audios & Demonstration Videos

Control Audio 1:  Control & Conquer - Cravings
Control Audio 2:  Control & Conquer - Feelings
Control Audio 3:  Control & Conquer - Self-Doubt & the Fear of Yo-Yo Dieting
Control Audio 4:  Control & Conquer - I Believe in Me/Once it's off I Keep it Off
Control Audio 5:  Control & Conquer – Overeating & Bingeing

## Program Audios & Demonstration Videos

Program Audio 1:        Eliminate Greedy Appetite
Program Audio 2:        Motivation to Move your Body & Exercise
Program Audio 3:        Be Stress Fee

## Rewire Audios

Rewire Audio 1: Rewire for Slim & Healthy Cardio Version - Unzip the Fat Suit

Rewire Audio 2: Rewire for Slim & Healthy Relax Version – Unzip the Fat Suit

Rewire Audio 3: Rewire for Confidence Cardio Version - Build Confidence & Self Esteem

Rewire Audio 4: Rewire for Confidence Relax Version – Build Confidence & Self Esteem

## CPR Mind Potential Kit PDF Strategies and Tools

- Map Your Progress Chart (Commitment 1)
- 10 Commitments Chart & 10 Commitments Reminder
- The Power of Three - Do 3 Things List
- Quick Cheat Sheet 1 (Control Cravings/Feelings Tapping Chart)
- Craving Buster Cheat Sheet 2 (Control Cravings/Feelings Tapping Chart)
- I AM chart

## YouTube Channel: *http://www.youtube.com/MaggieWilde*

There are also a number of *free* demonstration videos available on my YouTube channel. The videos have been designed to help you gain the most from the Control Tapping techniques. Please feel free to subscribe to *http://youtube.com/ MaggieWilde* for all the current demonstration videos and more as they are added in the future.

## What to Do – You can prepare by following these easy steps

Step 1: Download and save the CPR Kit to your personal device

Step 2: Begin using the audios and other strategies at appropriate stages of the book (I'll recommend certain audios as you go through the book)

Step 3: Use the *Program Audio* called: ***Eliminate Greedy Appetite*** – once a day for 5 days (you can start this today if you wish). Then alternate this audio with other *Program Audios* as often as you wish thereafter

Step 4: Use the *Control Audios and Videos* as and when you need them to control unhelpful emotions, resistance and cravings (this will be explained in Chapters 3 & 4)

Step 5:   Use the Rewire Audios once per day or as often as you choose

Step 6:   Alternate all other Audios as often as you wish

## Summary

- Start with the Program Audio: ***Eliminate Greedy Appetite*** once a day for a minimum of 5 days
- Alternate this with other *Program Audios* at least once per day for 31 days thereafter (some people enjoy them so much they never stop using them every now and then)
- Use the *Control Audios* daily as and when required to control cravings or unhelpful feelings and to build the belief in yourself that you can be slim and healthy permanently
- Use the *Rewire Audios*: Unzip the Fat Suit / Build Confidence as often as you wish (repetition is the key here, this will be explained later)
- Use the Program Audio: Be Stress Free as often as you wish to help you manage stress levels more effectively (the more relaxed you are about unzipping the fat suit, the more easily the fat suit comes off. The importance of this will be explained throughout the book.

*Enjoy the journey to find the slimmer and healthier you!*

# ONE

---

# The 5 Keys to Think Slim & Healthy – It's all in your mind

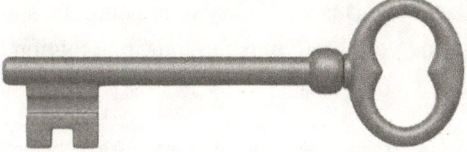

There are five keys that will help you achieve the success you desire. This chapter will explain those keys and outline how to use them in order to gain the most from the book and the CPR Mind Potential audios. Understanding these keys will help you implement the strategies and solutions in the book and the audios more effectively. They will help you control unhelpful thoughts, emotions and habits regarding your body and food. They will also help you lay the foundation and rewire more helpful thoughts, emotional states and actions.

There is a lot to absorb in this chapter; it will take a little effort on your behalf to do so, however the benefits to you will be life changing. I recommend you come back to this chapter if you need clarity to gain the most from the exercises in the book. Once you have an understanding of these keys, the remainder of the *unzip the fat suit* process will be so easy for you to put into practice. Your body, mind, spirit and your health will thank you for it. After absorbing this chapter, the exercises in the book, the Ten Commitments, the CPR audios and how to develop your motivational approach, will be much easier for you.

The CPR audios will work whether you read this chapter or not. However understanding the 5 Keys will make rewiring your brain for permanent slim and healthy easier. By absorbing the valuable information and using the skills outlined, the CPR audios, and strategies later in the book, will work even faster, meaning you'll unzip the fat suit more easily.

So take your time, absorb the outline of each key and email us if you need further explanation. info@thepotentialist.com

## The 5 Keys

❶ **Reality versus Imagination.** You were born with a brain that doesn't know the difference between real and imagined. This is the first key to unzipping the fat suit and rewiring for slim and healthy. We'll explain why soon.

❷ **Imagination.** You were born with an imagination – the ability to playact and pretend 'as if'. This is a vital key to creating the slim and healthy you from the inside. I'll guide you through using your imagination to gain maximum results.

❸ **Neuro-plasticity.** You were born with a brain that continues to develop new neural pathways (new memories, beliefs, reactions and skills) and learn new things, till the day you die.

> Science now tells us that the brain is able to adapt and change no matter how old we are. It says the brain is 'plastic', malleable, changeable and adaptable hence the science of Neuro-plasticity. In the case of a stroke for example, neuroplasticity can help other parts of the brain adapt or rewire alternative neural pathways that will by-pass the damaged area in order to relearn skills that may have been affected by the stroke. I will show you how to take advantage of your brain's natural ability to learn, adapt and develop.

> The science of neuroplasticity says the brain can continue to create new neural pathways (roadmaps/blueprints), clearer thinking, more appropriate emotional responses and stimulate different chemical and therefore emotional reactions, throughout your entire life. Once you know how to help your brain do this, nothing can stop you. This means changing unhelpful thoughts, feelings and habits and, rewiring better ones, is easier than you ever thought possible.

❹ **Two Processing Systems.** You were born with a brain that has two processing systems: conscious processing (short term memory, logic, reasoning, analysis, judgement, thinking) and subconscious processing (long term memory, habits and instincts, automatic responses such as digestion, breathing, hunger).

When these two systems operate in harmony we have balance. When they don't we have that dreaded internal conflict I mentioned in the Introduction. Thanks to Neuro-plasticity, I can now help you control, program and re-wire both processing systems effectively so they are working toward the same outcome. *(Eliminating internal conflict)*. This is one of the many reasons why the CPR audios and the strategies in the book are so important.

❺ **Conscious Analysis and Thinking.** As mentioned in Key 4, the conscious part of your mind is the thinking, analysing, judging and decision making part.

Using this part of your mind to critically analyse (and assess) is important for two reasons. *Firstly* the conscious part analyses your current experience and determines whether your subconscious reaction today is appropriate for you based on your goals and desires.

When you use conscious critical analysis, you can assess which thoughts, feelings and habits are not helping you anymore. Then CPR Mind Potential audios and other strategies throughout the book, help you activate Key 3 (Neuro-plasticity) to help you change what isn't working for you.

*Secondly,* you're ability to consciously analyse and think is important to help you discover your '*Why*', *(your Why is your motivating factor)*. When you are emotionally attached to 'Why' you want to be slim and healthy, you will feel more inspired to continue towards your unzip the fat suit goal.

Your '*Why*' is made up of the important benefits that you gain by achieving your goal, and the strength of your desire and your determination to do so. It also helps you assess what is working for you now, and how to reinforce that. This reasoning process will help you tailor your Ten Commitments (the plan), to suit your specific needs. (The Ten Commitments are outlined in Chapter 2).

## Key One Explained:

## Reality versus Imagination

It is vital to understand one very real truth about your brain –

***Your Brain does not know the difference between real & imagined***

## Mind Rehearsal

a) Your brain cannot distinguish between real or imagined. If you watch a horror movie, your body reacts with a physical stress response by increasing your heart rate and releasing adrenalin. Or in the case of a sad movie, it reacts by creating tears or emotional sensations. Even though you consciously know the movie is not real, your brain releases Neuro-chemicals that signal to your body to react as though it is.

Think about the last time you watched a horror, or an emotional movie. What instinctive response did your body have that you tried to control? Can you remember the last time you went to the cinema to watch a movie that had a 'sad' scene. If it wasn't you or one of your friends, there was someone in the audience trying to 'pretend' they weren't crying. This response happens because the subconscious 'believes' the tragedy is happening to you. The brain does not have the capacity to discern the difference between a movie and reality.

In fact, brain scans show that the brain is active, (neural pathways fire) in the same areas whether you are physically experiencing something, or mentally rehearsing and imagining it. (Restak, Richard, MD. *The New Brain*, p. 179. PA: Rodale, 2003.)

## Fun Exercise:

Close your eyes and imagine biting into your favourite fruit, make it a nice juicy one. Perhaps it's a delicious red, crisp, sweet apple or a mango or strawberry. Imagine or pretend as vividly as you can, as if you can taste, smell, sense and even feel the textures of the flesh, seeds, skin and pulp in your mouth now. Remember the smells associated with the fruit too. Perhaps you might recall or have an impression of the smell that lingered on your hands? Pretend as if that it is happening again now.

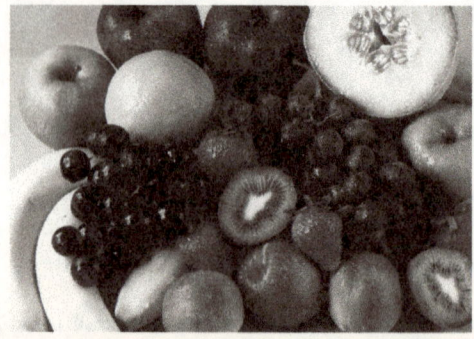

Did your saliva glands produce saliva? Did you experience an impression of textures, sensations or smells? Your level of response will be dependent upon the level of engagement you allowed your imagination to have. (Refer to Key 3). Your brain did not know the difference between imagining the fruit, and actually eating it. (Assuming you like fruit – if not, exchange fruit with your favourite food).

Elite athletes and highly successful people use their imagination to visualise in a similar targeted way to improve their results. When you mentally rehearse a successful outcome, your brain creates and strengthens appropriate neural pathways (memory circuitry) to achieve it. This happens because the brain now has a memory that it thinks is real. In the case of the athlete, the brain assumes that the athlete already knows how to be successful, because the rehearsed neural pathways already exist.

For the purposes of unzipping the fat suit, when you *mind rehearse* slim and healthy actions, the brain circuitry that is required to help you make healthier choices, or to get out of bed and go for that walk, now exist.

The actions are no longer as foreign to the brain, so after repeatedly mind rehearsing this, you are more likely to choose the healthier option next time. Once something has been rehearsed enough in the mind, the brain knows which chemicals to release in order to stimulate the right level of motivation. The brain understands which messages to send to the limbs, muscles and organs to make the desired outcomes happen more easily.

*In other words, the brain didn't know that your mental rehearsal was not real. It fired the same neurons, which stimulated the same chemical releases, which fired the same muscles in the body, as if the movement was indeed taking place. That is why you will have experienced some level of response when thinking about eating your favourite fruit in the previous exercise.*

No matter what outcome you aim for, the way to achieve it permanently, is to deliberately, and with conscious input, choose to **program and rewire** your mind by:

1. Finding clarity about your goal, why you want it and the benefits you will experience when you have it *(Your 'Why')*
2. Following a plan *(The 10 Commitments – Chapter 2)*
3. *Using your imagination to mind rehearse* your desired outcomes, as if they are already real by using the *CPR audios and other strategies* provided

31

4.  Adding ***heightened positive emotions*** while mind rehearsing. (Pretending 'as if' or faking the successful outcome in your mind, as if it's real now)
5.  Using ***Repetition***. Repeating the process until your brain has a 'memory' (*neural pathway or blueprint map*) of the outcome you want

**This is why, when you use the following formula, you unzip the fat suit permanently.**

1.  ***Ten Commitments (chapter 2)*** +
2.  **CPR – Control, Program and Rewire audios** +
3.  **Mind Rehearsal.** Imagine your ideal weight, shape and size as if it's real now *(Do this repeatedly and add positive 'feelings'/ heightened sensations*

---

*"We can achieve any realistic goal if we keep on thinking of that goal, and stop thinking any negative thoughts about it." Napoleon Hill*

---

It is important to note that different people *imagine or 'Mind Rehearse'* differently. Some people see the image in their mind, some people feel it or sense it, and some people get an impression or even hear it. The more senses and emotions (such as excitement or gratitude) you activate while doing the mind rehearsal, the more successful the outcome. Simply pretend if you have to at first.

## Key Two:

## Imagination

As very young children we were naturally able, and without inhibition, to access a deep creative imagination. This ability allowed us to pretend or act 'as if' things were real, when sometimes they were not.

Did you or someone you knew play imaginary games as a child? Games like 'cowboys and Indians', 'teacher and student', 'selling at the store'? Did you or your friends have pretend tea parties with your childhood teddy bears or dolls?

This natural talent, the imagination, is developed at a time in childhood when we begin to act 'as if' things are real (between the ages of 2 to 7 years). As adults, we forget that we still have that ability, or we feel 'silly', too grown up to playact anymore. For the purpose of unzipping the fat suit using your mind, the more you reactivate this ability, the faster your results will be. So have fun with it and be a kid again. Play the 'skinny' game as if it was real, and your brain will eventually learn that it is.

I want you to approach mind rehearsal and the CPR audios with fun, imagination and a carefree attitude. Put your critical thinking aside while you listen, and just 'pretend' you're already at your goal.

'Play-acting' is essential to the development and imprinting of deep neural pathways (a new slim and healthy map) that will help your brain learn. Children use their imagination without holding anything back; role-playing helps their brains develop neural pathways that store knowledge about how to behave, respond and perceive the world, and how to exist and interact within it. Roleplaying and acting 'as if', is drawing upon your brain's 'plasticity' to learn.

While using CPR audios and Mind Rehearsal techniques your brain will develop new neural connections associated with slim and healthy. When you use your imagination to pretend like a child with a carefree attitude, your brain will use this process to create 'memory circuitry'. When listening to the CPR audios and when doing Mind Rehearsal it is important to re-kindle that natural ability to 'pretend' or 'play-act'. You did it naturally as a child; you can do it again now.

**Your role, if you should choose to take it, is to have fun. It is to play, make believe, imagine and pretend the healthy actions, images, thoughts and feelings I suggest in the audios, are already real – right here and right now.**

*Your only limit is your imagination - imagine it, and it is so.*

## Key Three:

## Neuro-plasticity – How your brain learns

For the purposes of unzipping the fat suit permanently, I have outlined 5 ways your brain learns (develops new neural pathways – new 'memories' or 'maps'). When you use these skills, your brain learns these new 'maps' faster.

## 5 WAYS IN WHICH YOUR BRAIN LEARNS

| | |
|---|---|
| **1** | **Our brain learns and imprints new neural pathways based on what we are taught by authority figures and people we value, respect or fear**<br><br>*What we learn from authority figures is more likely to be accepted as truth, especially when we are young.*<br><br>***Example 1****: You fell over and hurt yourself. You learned that sweets or biscuits were comforting because Granny, (who you respected and loved) made it all better with a biscuit and a cuddle. Somehow when Granny gave you the biscuit and cuddle, the pain was minimised.*<br><br>*Example 2: You were taught that you have to eat everything on the plate. Your parents said, "it's naughty not to finish everything" or "there are starving kids in Ethiopia, so eat it and be grateful".* |
| **2** | **Our brain learns when we identify with a group**<br><br>*If society or our community or peers say it is so, we learn to believe and accept it.*<br><br>*Example 1: Mob rule - sporting events and war times where group energy provides identification. People often behave in ways and believe things that they normally wouldn't.*<br><br>*Example 2: You learned as a young person that smoking, drinking alcohol or 'wagging' school was cool. Your friends all did it, and you felt a sense of belonging when you did too.* |

**3**

**Our brain learns (develops deep neural pathways) when we experience intense Positive and or Negative Emotions, Sensory States and Feelings**

*Intense emotional states, feelings or strong physical sensations can open the doorway for the brain to 'learn'. While our conscious mind is focused on the emotion or feeling, our sub-conscious imprints deep neural connections (new maps in the brain) it learned from the intense experience. The conscious mind creates a perception about it (a judgement), as good or bad, based on the type of emotion experienced.*

*Importantly the subconscious does not differentiate between good or bad sensations or emotions. It is the **strength** of the emotion or sensation that causes strong electrical currents (new maps), to fire in the brain.*

***Example 1:*** *Remember Granny and the biscuit? You learned a 'new map' very quickly in a heightened emotional state that the 'hurt feeling' went away because the biscuit made you forget the pain and feel loved. You connected granny's cuddle and the biscuit with, 'I feel loved'. Later it simply became the 'biscuit' that replaced the cuddle. That's how the young brain interpreted it, and eventually it became a 'map' and then a 'truth'.*

***The long-term subconscious learning****: sugar, biscuit or something sweet - makes me feel - good, loved, safe or better.*

***Example 2****: Remember the starving kids in Ethiopia? You learned very quickly that you 'have to eat everything on the plate' while thinking of and feeling 'bad' for those 'starving kids'. At the same time perhaps, you were also feeling rebellious about 'having to eat everything on the plate' when you didn't really want to, didn't like it, or were already full.*

***The long-term subconscious 'map' learning****: I have to eat everything on my plate or other people will feel bad, I will get into trouble, I'm ungrateful or I am a naughty, bad person if I don't.*

| 4 | **Our brain learns (develops neural pathways, 'maps') through repetition.** By itself repetition is a relatively slow way to learn. However when heightened emotional states, feelings or sensations are added to the repetitive message, then the learning (map) is enhanced tremendously. |
|---|---|
| | If a child heard regularly that they were 'useless, hopeless, a greedy guts or naughty', and those repetitive comments made him or her feel bad, then the heightened emotional state they experienced when they heard these comments, ensured that the inappropriate learning was established quickly, perhaps, even becoming a limiting belief. |
| | **The Long-term subconscious learning**: "I must be unworthy, greedy, hopeless". As a result, this limiting belief, or some variation of it, is established. |
| | In the same way, if we create heightened positive states and provide clear healthy, confident messages, we can develop more helpful beliefs: |
| | **The long-term subconscious learning becomes**: "I am worthy, healthy, slim". |
| | This is one of the key reasons why the CPR audios work. With regular use of the audios, your brain absorbs the new way of thinking about your body, confidence and health. A new healthy 'map' is created. |
| | All while you relax back and engage in heightened positive emotional states. Acting 'as if' you have already achieved slim and healthy, creates the change faster. |
| 5 | Your brain develops neural pathways and learns when rhythm is included in the processes above. |
| | When a rhythm or a hypnotic heartbeat is used during the learning process, the learning (new map) is established even faster. |
| | I have created the CPR audios with the required rhythm to enhance learning. |

| | |
|---|---|
| **3 - 5 used together** | **Learning and developing neural pathways with CPR Audios and Mind Rehearsal**<br><br>*The fastest route to unzip the fat suit is to control, program and rewire your subconscious for the healthy slim you by combining steps 3 to 5.*<br><br>*Learning is enhanced (new maps in the brain are formed) when we do these steps:*<br><br>1. Find clarity on your desired outcome and your 'why' (why you want to achieve your goal)<br><br>2. Use the CPR Audios to Mind Rehearse the successful outcome<br><br>3. Use Repetition (do it again and again)<br><br>4. Add emotions, feelings and strong sensations while using the CPR audios and mind rehearsal tools (to achieve faster outcomes – feel it 'as if' it is real already)<br><br>5. Include rhythm (the hypnotic heart beat used in the CPR audio programs subliminally supports the suggestions and enhances learning).<br><br>***The Formula for Permanent Change therefore is:***<br><br>   • ***Make the decision to achieve Slim & Healthy +***<br>   • ***Emotionally Connect to 'Why' Do You Want it +***<br>   • ***Follow a Plan (The Ten Commitments) +***<br>   • ***Use CPR Audios & Mind Rehearsal +***<br>   • ***Add Feelings/sensations +***<br>   • ***Do it again and again +***<br>   • ***Enjoy the Rhythm***<br><br>        ***= Permanent Change***<br><br>*This is why those who use this formula and include my CPR audio technology, describe the change as, "the easiest thing they have ever done."* |

# Key Four

## Two Processing Systems

**Our mind processes on two levels – consciously and subconsciously.**

Your mind has two processing systems that help determine your behaviors and actions.

You make decisions, think, judge and analyse with the conscious processing part of your mind. However, the subconscious part controls your habits and automatic reactions, physical processes and all of the systems within your body such as breathing, heart rate, hormonal responses and digestion.

The subconscious part of your mind, importantly for the purpose of this book, also controls your sensations of hunger or fullness. For some of us, the subconscious may have been programmed with unhelpful emotional connections to food or eating too. For example it may have developed a connection between anger or loneliness, and sweets or chocolate.

The CPR audios will take your brain on a journey to a relaxed place that hovers between two brainwave states. These states are called self-hypnosis and meditation; they are the states that enhance learning. These states will happen automatically when you use the audios. In these states, the guided suggestions provided in the audios will help you mind rehearse the new healthy outcomes. In this way, you automatically program and rewire your brain for slim and healthy. In these states you can communicate directly with the subconscious part of your mind to create more appropriate behaviors and reactions.

These two brainwave states are the learning states. Self-hypnosis takes place in a brainwave state called 'Theta'. It is the place where the subconscious part of your mind operates. Meditation takes place in a brainwave state called 'Alpha' this is where your mind is inwardly focused and relaxation flows. In both these states your brain learns more effectively.

To understand the simplicity of how this works, I have provided a chart to outline the different brainwave states where learning and change (programming and rewiring new maps) is most likely to occur.

Our brain activity constantly moves between four natural brainwave states. These states are called: beta, alpha, theta and delta.

## Brainwave States

| Brainwave State | Level of Consciousness | What this means to you |
|---|---|---|
| **BETA** | • Awake<br>• Alert<br>• Conscious | Talking, higher levels would be excitement, argument, animation, stress or tension |
| **ALPHA** | • Relaxed Meditation<br>• Internal awareness and focus<br>• Conscious re-wiring/learning state | Calm and composed relaxed state of being, light meditation states, great for the Control and Rewiring audios |
| **THETA** | • Self-Hypnosis state<br>• Subconscious programming and rewiring/a deeper learning state<br>• Healing state<br>• Parasympathetic nervous system active in rest and digest<br>• Rapid Eye Movement (REM) | Deep tranquillity, calm. Extreme ability to focus your attention in specific areas. Lose track of time. For example: time disappears when you are watching a movie, reading, doing art or gardening. When you drive and don't remember the whole trip. You enter this state when using my Program & Rewire audios. It often seem as though time stands still. Deep day-dream state, drowsiness |
| **DELTA** | • Sleep<br>• Conscious processing inactive<br>• Sub-conscious processing is active | Various states of sleep. The conscious mind has gone to sleep, the subconscious is actively breathing, digesting, healing the body while the conscious part of you sleeps. |

The Meditative state of Alpha and the Self-Hypnosis state of Theta are the brain-wave states where learning happens more effectively. These are the states of mind that the CPR audios automatically guide you to.

Often as you attempt to program and rewire your mind for healthier outcomes, you can experience internal conflict about the outcome, or be distracted by the conscious mind interrupting or judging. You may want to be slim and healthy, but you subconsciously keep having cravings for chocolate or lack motivation to exercise. Often it can feel as though you are at odds with what you really want. In fact there can be an underlying subconscious program (previous map or blueprint) at play that needs to be updated or changed.

To help this update take place, I will briefly address the mind's two processing systems: the conscious system of critical awareness (conscious thought), and the subconscious system of automatic processes, thoughts and behaviours (unconscious reactions, thinking and systems of the body).

## The Processing Systems of the Conscious Mind

The conscious mind is often explained with the analogy of 'the tip of the iceberg'. The conscious mind is the part of the iceberg you see above the surface of the water. The subconscious on the other hand is the part of your mind that operates below the level of your normal consciousness. In the iceberg analogy, the subconscious mind is the more substantial part, under the water.

According to some theories the conscious mind only represents about 10 -12% of the potential of our mind. The subconscious represents the remaining 88-90%.

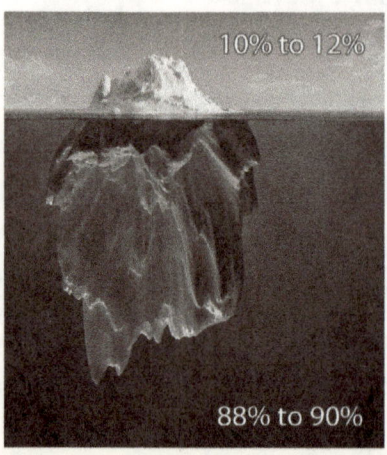

The conscious mind is mainly active when we are awake and is responsible for our decision-making, judgments, rationalisations and analysis. It only has *short-term memory* capacity and therefore mainly deals with the 'here and now'.

One of the aims of using the CPR audios is to help the conscious mind become *less attentive*. When using the audios some people will be aware of everything and others will drift in and out.

## The Subconscious Mind

The subconscious mind on the other hand, could be compared to the 'hard drive' of your computer. The information in the subconscious could be likened to the software driving the computer (you). The subconscious stores everything that has ever happened, every event, experience, reaction and our perceptions to it all. It stores our beliefs and instincts that help us determine what is wrong or right, and our instinctual emotional reactions and habits are programmed here too.

It controls our *Autonomic Nervous System (ANS)* such as the functions of our heartbeat, our lungs breathing, and all our other organs and systems of the body. Importantly it controls our hormonal system, our digestive system, our levels of hunger or satisfaction and thirst.

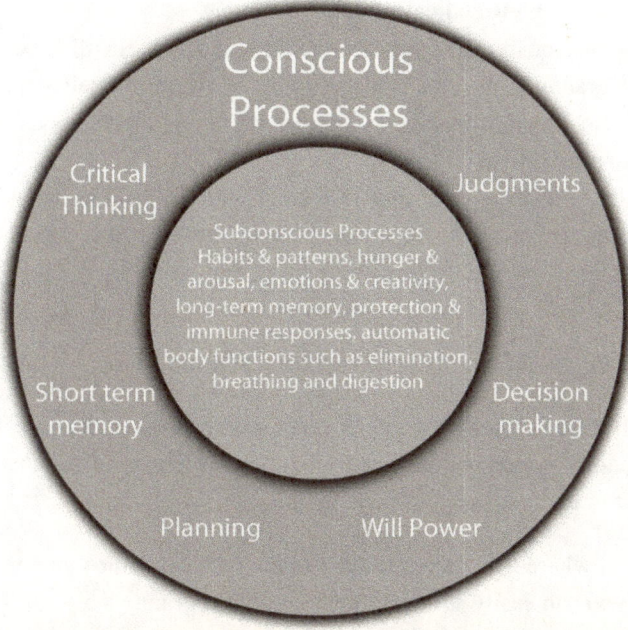

Unlike the conscious mind however, the subconscious has *no reasoning ability.* It's the part of our mind that doesn't understand the difference between real and imagined.

If you have consciously made a decision that sugary foods are 'bad' because your goal is to be slim and healthy, but your subconscious mind does not judge that sugary foods are 'bad', then internal conflict happens. *Remember Granny and the biscuit/cuddle?* Your subconscious doesn't understand your conscious mind's new objective yet, so it still operates under the premise that "biscuits make you feel better" because they always did.

Until the CPR audios have helped your subconscious learn that biscuits or sugary foods are no longer appropriate for you and no longer desired, then it will continue to respond with your old habit. It will continue to stimulate the neural pathways that cause cravings for something sweet, whenever you feel hurt or wounded.

That's when the 're-education' or 'rewiring' of your subconscious minds' blue-print, your map, becomes imperative. This is achieved by using the strategies in the book and the CPR audios.

**Scenario:**

- You decide to unzip the fat suit and need to change a few unhealthy habits
- Alas! Your subconscious doesn't know this yet because you haven't listened to the CPR audios enough
- You consciously want to unzip the fat suit, but you still subconsciously crave granny's sweet biscuit when you feel hurt or lonely
- You also still subconsciously eat everything on the plate even when you are already full
- Until you use the CPR audios enough, the desire for granny's 'sweet' comfort still persists. No matter how frustrated you are, the 'map' still exists and the cravings will continue

**This is where the 'C' of the CPR audios comes into play.**

The C = Control and Conquer, which is exactly what these audios do. They control the automatic response of the past so that you *interrupt* the automatic pattern (your 'map' or neural pathway) in your brain.

- This is where it is important to use the Control audios and exercises so that you can easily say no to the craving for granny's biscuit.

- At the same time, use the *program and rewire* audios daily to help you re-*educate (lay the foundation of the new map that stimulates different reactions)* permanently.
- *Control audios* save your butt in the event of an inappropriate craving or urge, they do this by interrupting the neural pathway that causes the craving. *Control audios* are like your 'emergency kit'.
- *Program and rewire* audios lay the foundation of the new healthy reaction (map), and through repetition, change the habitual response permanently. Yeah!
- Eventually, after using the *program and rewire* audios enough, you won't need the *control audios* at all.
- After using the CPR audios often enough too, the cravings won't happen and you will be in control *consciously and subconsciously,* to choose slim and healthy responses.

---

*It becomes automatic! The battle is won; you are no longer fighting with yourself internally! Your conscious and subconscious processes are aligned with your healthier goals! You are able to unzip the fat suit with ease!*

---

## Key Five:

## Conscious Analysis & Thinking

An important key in creating the slim and healthy change you desire is to have a strong and valid reason 'Why'. It is vital that you use conscious analysis to regularly assess: *"Why do I want to unzip the fat suit? Why do I want to be slim and healthy?"*

Once you are *emotionally connected* to the benefits of unzipping the fat suit, then you are well on the way to creating it, because that's how your brain learns. *(Emotionally connected means when you contemplate your goal, you experience physical sensations and /or you feel eager, happy, excited and even look forward to it with eager anticipation).*

### 'Why' Do You want to be Slim and Healthy?
### What are Your Motivating Factors?

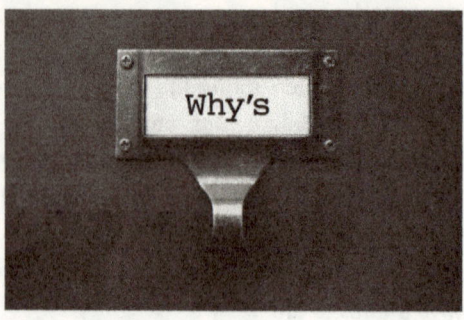

To discover your 'Why', it is important to ask yourself these questions - be as honest as you can:

| Your *'WHY'S* – are your *Motivating Factors*<br>Why Do you Want to Unzip the Fat Suit Permanently? | |
| --- | --- |
| **What benefits will I experience once I unzip the fat suit and achieve slim and healthy?**<br><br>**This is your 'Why' so make it really mean something to you. Why do you want to become slim and healthy?**<br><br>**Why is it important to me? How will my life be different when I am slim and healthy? Sell it to yourself!**<br><br>*(Ensure these benefits are solution focused not problem focused. For example – I won't puff as much climbing stairs is problem focused. It focuses on the old problem of 'being out of breath'. Whereas - I breathe easily when I climb stairs is solution focused. It focuses on 'breathing easily'. The examples I have given in the adjacent box are solution focused)* | **The benefits I experience are…**<br><br>(*E.g.* I will climb stairs and breathe easily, I can have energy to travel more, more energy with kids, live longer to see kids grow up, wear jeans comfortably, feel healthier, be comfortable in a bikini/ swimmers) |

*(continued)*

| | |
|---|---|
| **On a scale of 0 to 10 how important are each of these benefits / 'Whys'? Rate each one.** | |
| **Which benefits / 'Whys' rate the highest on that scale of 0 to 10?**<br><br>**Which ones create strong sensations or emotions when you think about achieving them?**<br><br>The highest ones are the key benefits, the 'Whys' to focus on when using the audio programs (the most important reason or reasons for choosing to be slim and healthy) | |

If you haven't been able to establish strong emotional connections to your benefits or 'Whys' as yet, ask yourself these questions:

1. When will being slim and healthy be important to me?

2. Am I holding onto the fat suit based on fears or doubts such as:

- **Who will I be without the fat suit?**
- **What if I fail? What will people think if I fail?**
- **I doubt that I can do it or**
- **I've tried to do it before and put it all back on**

If this is the case, congratulations for being honest with yourself. Keep reading because the book and the audios will help you address these unhelpful issues, doubts and fears.

*This book is definitely for you, you are one of the reasons I wrote it.*

Simply keep reading, use the CPR audios (even if you don't believe the slim and healthy suggestions at the moment – use them anyway – fake it till you make it!). Come back to this chapter and reassess your benefits and 'Whys' every now and then as you read the book.

If you haven't yet established a strong, healthy, emotionally connected '*Why*', don't be concerned right now. Using the CPR audios to establish and release any potential underlying patterns that have kept you stuck in the fat suit will help resolve this. The CPR audios have been designed to help you shift these, if they are there.

All you need to do right now is to focus on the '*Whys*' when I ask you to, and as often as you wish. Pretend them for the moment and regularly reassess your 'Whys'. **The 'Whys' are your compass**.

Use your '*Whys*' when you are directed to in the mind rehearsal parts of the audios. The new neural pathway connections (maps) will get stronger as you repeatedly use them.

In the following chapter I address your plan, the important Ten Commitments. I have briefly mentioned them before, but now it's time to delve into the solutions, the 'How' do I unzip the fat suit permanently.

# Two

---

## Program the Ten Commitments – Your Plan

### The Secret to Your Success

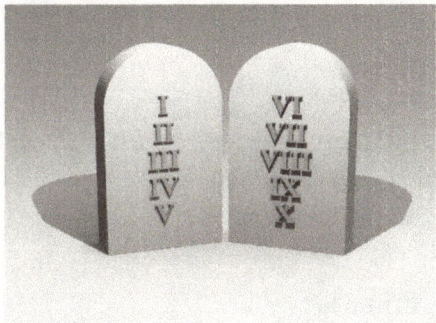

In order to unzip the fat suit permanently, it is important to have a plan.

Research shows that people who plan and make themselves accountable to that plan, are far more successful in achieving their goals. Professor Richard Wiseman in his book *59 Seconds – Think a Little Change a Lot,* outlines a research study with 5000 people from around the world. Many people in the study decided their goal was to lose weight.

He discovered that only 10 % of participants achieved their goal, and *all* of those that did, had a definite plan. They developed a step-by-step strategy and then broke their goal into lots of smaller "goals".

### *They had a PLAN*

These 10 Commitments are your plan. Those who follow this 10-step plan, achieve their ideal weight, shape and size every time.

## Fool Proof Commitments

The 10 Commitments are fool proof. The more you carry out the commitments, the more the commitments become automatic for you.

Using the CPR audios is one of the commitments. Remember the audios help your subconscious mind control, program and rewire your thoughts, feelings and habits. However, another benefit to the audios is that the 10 Commitments are woven into them. So the more you listen to the audios, the more likely you are to do the commitments, and the more you do the commitments, the more likely you are to do the audios. Voila! A fool proof plan!

**By doing the 10 Commitments daily you will:**

- Reduce weight easily
- Create healthier habits and behaviour
- Build self-confidence
- Increase motivation
- Develop personal responsibility to yourself and your body
- Become a better friend to yourself
- Keep the weight off permanently

**These commitments will also help you:**

- Disconnect any past unhealthy relationships with food and eating
- Maximise your weight reduction in a healthy, permanent way
- Create new positive habits
- Increase your desire for healthy options and smaller portions
- Activate your ability to choose slim and healthy automatically

Repetition helps your brain learn, so I ask that you use these 10 Commitments *every day.* Use them until one day they happen naturally for you.

---

*These 10 commitments, the strategies in the book and the CPR audios are the SECRET TO YOUR SUCCESS.*

---

Once you've achieved your ideal weight, size and shape, the commitments are easily adapted to help you maintain your slimmer body. You will have become slim and healthy, and slim and healthy will have become you.

If you want permanent success then I urge you to please take these commitments seriously, commit to do them daily. Those that do this, achieve their goals every time. As a subconscious reinforcement, once you agree to each commitment, please sign where indicated.

## COMMITMENT ONE

### Map your Progress & Mind Rehearse Your Goal Outfit

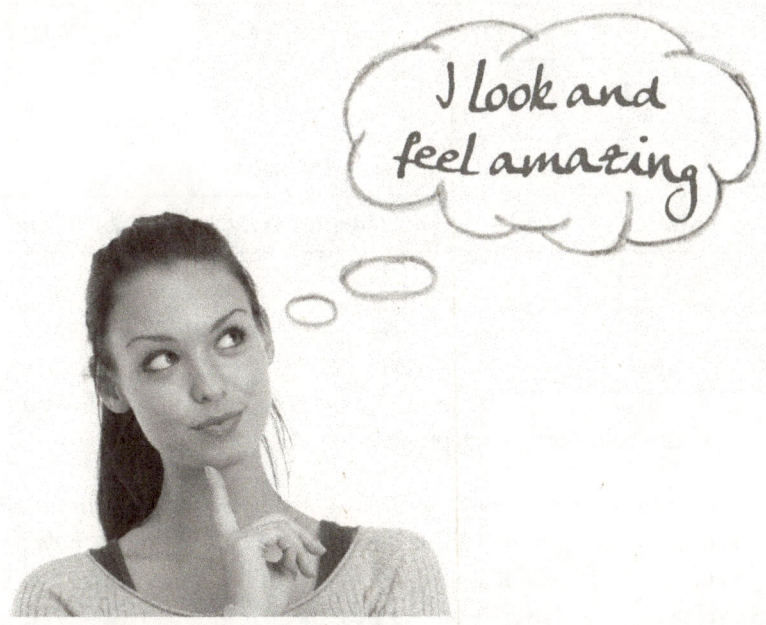

**Step 1:** Complete the 'Map Your Progress' chart provided, set small chunk goals. At each level set a realistic clothing size and weight

**Step 2:** Buy something new in your first level goal size. Make it something you really want to wear, but don't try it on

**Step 3:** Mind rehearse wearing that new outfit everyday

# MAP YOUR PROGRESS CHART

| First Goal Size and Weight | | | |
|---|---|---|---|
| **Current Size** | **Goal Size** | **Current Weight** | **Goal Weight** |
|  |  |  |  |

| Second Goal Size and Weight | | | |
|---|---|---|---|
| **Current Size** | **Goal Size** | **Current Weight** | **Goal Weight** |
|  |  |  |  |

| Third Goal Size and Weight | | | |
|---|---|---|---|
| **Current Size** | **Goal Size** | **Current Weight** | **Goal Weight** |
|  |  |  |  |

| Fourth Goal Size and Weight | | | |
|---|---|---|---|
| **Current Size** | **Goal Size** | **Current Weight** | **Goal Weight** |
|  |  |  |  |

Once you have achieved that first level, do this process again and focus on the next goal size as a completely fresh program.

**Tip:** Be realistic in your first level weight and size. Your success will be easier when you consider your goal believable or possible at first. If you are now a size 20 and you buy a size 10 pair of knickers as your goal outfit, you may not be able to *believe* yet that you will ever be able to wear them. At this early stage, the goal size must seem achievable in the not too distant future. So I encourage you to buy a goal outfit one or two sizes smaller than you are wearing now.

Once you are able to wear the first goal outfit comfortably, then focus on your next level goal, and buy a new outfit in that new second level goal size.

*N.B. your goal outfit does not need to be expensive. It can be as simple as a t-shirt or a pair of knickers. It's the size and the desire to wear it that is important, rather than the cost.*

Regularly achieving smaller goals will provide the evidence to your brain that you are successful. The more your mind gets used to success, the more it is likely to help you achieve it again.

I have already discussed the importance of mind rehearsal and imagination as part of the 5 keys. I explained that this natural ability is effective because your mind does not know the difference between real and imagined. As part of Commitment One, I ask you to draw upon that skill to imagine or pretend that you already fit into this new outfit easily. In fact, you may even wish to imagine how it would feel if it was a little too big for you already.

When there is something you want and you behave in a way that indicates you already have achieved it, your mind will assume you already do. It will do everything it can to direct your attention to that outcome. So act 'as if' your body is already wearing that first level goal outfit comfortably. Once you can actually wear it, buy something new in the next realistic goal size.

Continue this process until you reach your ideal weight, shape and size.

**There are guidelines to purchase this outfit:**

- The outfit must be NEW, not something you already have in the wardrobe. If it is something that you no longer fit into, there will be disappointment attached to it. If there are unhelpful associations to the outfit such as 'I can't fit into it anymore' or 'I wish I hadn't put the weight on' or 'what a waste', then the subconscious has to delete those unhelpful feelings and thoughts before it can refocus your mind and emotions on how wonderful it will be to wear it.
- When your goal outfit has no history attached, you create positive anticipation about it. This way your mind can rewire by rehearsing wearing it each day.
- It doesn't have to be expensive, but it must be something you really want to wear.
- Hang the outfit where you can see it often, even perhaps photograph it and use it as wallpaper on your computer or phone.
- Mind rehearse *as if you already wear it comfortably, perhaps it's already a little too big.*
- Engage all of your senses in that mind rehearsal experience. Pretend you can feel the fabric, imagine the places you would wear it as if those events, places and people are real now.
- First thing in the morning look at your outfit and mind rehearse wearing it.

- Last thing at night look at it and mind rehearse wearing it.
- Imagine it at different times throughout the day (use any spare minute to imagine how wearing your new outfit will feel).

Remember you don't need to believe it yet, simply pretend it if you have to. The outcome you are programming is for the brain and body to become used to feeling slimmer, wearing smaller clothes, feeling healthier and behaving with more confidence. The more you practice and pretend this; the easier the journey to slim and healthy will be for you.

Once you have filled out your 'map your progress' chart, and you are ready to commit to buying your first level outfit and to mind rehearse wearing it, sign here:

**Signature:**                                              **Date:**

## COMMITMENT TWO

# Listen to CPR – Mind Potential audios daily

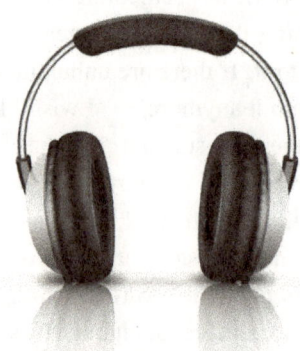

- As repetition is one of the ways the brain learns, then using one or more of the audios every day is vital.
- The first audio for repetitive reprogramming is: **Eliminate Greedy Appetite**. If you haven't started listening to it yet, then begin today. Continue for 5 days at least once per day. After this, mix and match listening to the other audios as you wish. Rotate it from day 6 onwards with the other audios.

- It is essential that you listen to it at least once a day (preferably twice at first). Remember the audio will lay the foundation for new neural pathways that will change your association and attitude towards your body, food and exercise. It will reinforce each of the 10 Commitments to help make them automatic.

Remember when you first learned to drive? At first you had to think about doing it consciously, perhaps making mistakes, but eventually it became automatic for you. You no longer needed to think consciously about how much pressure to apply to the brakes to pull up at traffic lights, or what route to take home.

Once you'd done it a number of times, you did it automatically. The same thing will begin to take place with the commitments. You will begin to do them on autopilot.

- You will increase the audio's effects if you listen using headphones
- When you use the CPR audios regularly re-assess your 'Why's'. Think about the benefits you will experience at your ideal weight, shape and size
- Sit in a comfortable chair or rest on your bed or sofa listening to the suggestions
- It's okay to drift off every now or then, however do attempt to hear each new audio with a semi-conscious awareness at least a few times when you first start

**NB: It is very important that you never listen to the audios while driving or operating machinery**.

Once you are ready to commit to use the CPR audios daily, sign here:

**Signature:**                                                **Date:**

## COMMITMENT THREE

## Weigh Only Once Per Week

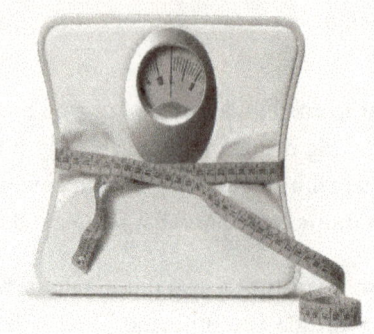

It is very important that you commit to only check your official progress by weighing in once per week.

Some people become obsessed with the weigh in process, so it is important that I address this issue. Body weight can fluctuate on a daily or hourly basis. If you weigh in more than once per week, you might experience unhelpful emotions if the numbers on the scale fluctuate from one day to the next.

Body weight will slightly vary for many natural reasons. It is influenced by whether you drank enough water, or whether your body stored extra fluids to cope with issues such as alcohol or toxins. It reflects whether you have evacuated your bowels or perspired. Whether you have eaten or exercised. It is indicative of what you are wearing, and even fluctuates with hormonal issues. For women in particular, it will fluctuate based on what time of the month it is too.

If you weigh in more than once per week, you do not give the body time to adjust to *actual fat loss*. It will only reflect the natural fluctuations in fluid, food, waste, digestion and hormones.

I consulted with a client who was addicted to weighing herself four, sometimes five times per day. Her mind was obsessed with every mouthful of food and every drink. She would weigh herself before the toilet, after the toilet, before a walk and after. She weighed first thing in the morning and often last thing at night. Each week she would come to the sessions more depressed. The excess weight was coming off, however the progress was slower than average. She confirmed she was following the commitments … all except this one!

When you repeatedly weigh in *and* experience heightened feelings of stress based on what the scales might or might not show, then your subconscious learns quickly that your weight, food, water and everything else is to be feared. The more you stress about this, the harder it becomes to reduce weight.

The disappointment this client experienced every day, led her to feel more unworthy and helpless about achieving her goal *(even though she was losing weight)*.

The highs and lows became confusing for her body too. It was as though the numbers on the scale controlled her emotions. This led to hopeless and helpless feelings. Each week I had to inspire her to dig herself out of a hole deeper than the week before, even though she had dropped over a kilogram.

One of the most significant issues with weighing in more than once per week is that we are pandering to our need for instant gratification. Many of us have become hooked on needing to know, have, do everything NOW. The media teases us with *'Buy now and pay later'* or *'24 months interest free, we'll deliver it today'*.

Often why we have put on weight in the first place, is as a result of fulfilling this need for instant gratification. We see chocolate cake and want the satisfaction now.

**Do you ever finish everything on the plate even though you were satisfied way before the plate was clean?**

I often hear clients say, *"Ooh I couldn't leave any, it was just too yummy"* or *"I was worried that there wasn't going to be any left for me later?"*

One of the ways to deal with *instant gratification syndrome* is to remember *"I can always do it /have it another time"*. When you diffuse the need to have it or do it NOW, you can remember that you live in a world of plenty. There's always more if you need it one day. There's always tomorrow, you don't have to have or do it all today.

The same applies to weighing in. The scales are not going to disappear. They will still be there tomorrow and next week and the week after. The solution comes from learning how to build anticipation.

In our fast food, fast living world where everything happens TODAY, we have overlooked the fact that looking forward to something provides far greater joy. Rather than feeling disappointed that it's all gone, we can feel safe that there's more to look forward to if we ever need it.

When you respond to the need for instant gratification, you are often left with the guilt or shame that you ate too much, or the regret that: *'If I'd waited till the end of the week, the results would have been better'*.

When you experience this constant upheaval, your brain learns that your weight is something to fear or dread. It learns that the number on the scales controls how you feel and what you think. It often controls your behaviour too, because if you have an emotional connection where disappointment leads to binge eating, or doing well leads to reward eating (*'I did well, so I can reward myself with a treat'*), then you end up back on the merry-go-round of yo-yo dieting.

**Once you are ready to commit to choose your weigh in day and weigh only once per week, sign here:**

**Signature:**                                                    **Date:**

## COMMITMENT FOUR

### Rewire Digestion - Chew Slowly - Chew Each Mouthful Consciously/Mindfully

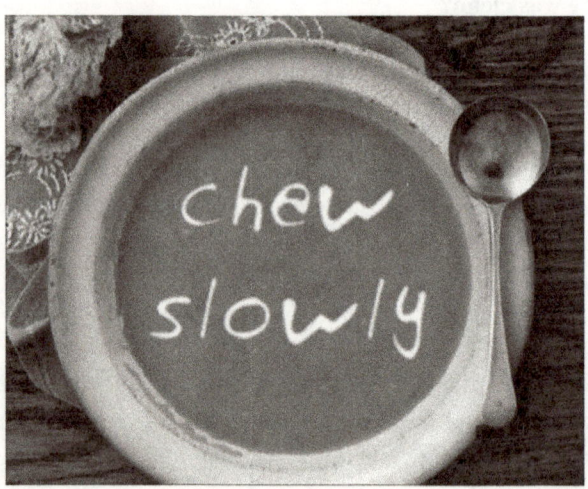

Do you inhale food; is fast food becoming faster food? Many people eat on the run. Busy lives mean they squeeze their meals into busy parts of the day. Some people eat in the car on the way to work, some while at the computer or while doing other things.

This commitment is about eating more mindfully, enjoying your food more and in a more relaxed way. This commitment however, is also about slowing the speed at which you eat and chew. In fact, I ask that you now consciously chew each mouthful thoroughly (approximately 15-30 times per mouthful).

This commitment is so important in your unzip the fat suit journey that I have dedicated Chapter 8 to the topic. In that chapter, I focus on the connection between stress and chewing, and the role that plays in how much weight you lose, your ability to digest food, and the speed at which you unzip the fat suit.

Research has proven that those who chew between 20-30 times or more for each mouthful, are slimmer. So look out for why and how in Chapter 8.

All I ask now is that you make a commitment to yourself that you will begin to enjoy every mouthful more, saviour the food. Start to focus and enjoy the texture of the food, the flavours and smells as you chew. Think and feel positively about the food you are eating and of course, do it more slowly.

When you do this, you experience more pleasure in the eating process. When your focus shifts from quantity to quality, from speed to savour, you automatically begin to eat less.

Remember the CPR audios help to program and rewire your mind to make chewing more slowly, automatic for you.

**Once you feel ready to commit to chewing more consciously / mindfully and to read Chapter 8, please accept this commitment:**

**Signature:**                                                    **Date:**

## COMMITMENT FIVE

**Push your plate away as soon as you feel comfortable – Check in to your stomach for the satisfied feeling**

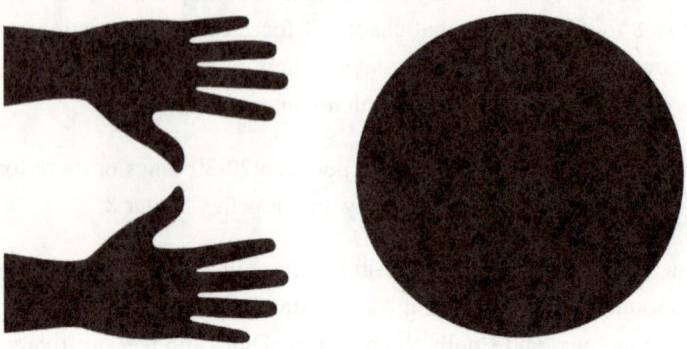

This commitment is focused on learning how to activate, recognise and respond to the full and satisfied feeling. The importance of 'listening' to your stomach and pausing between mouthfuls, allows you to 'check in' with the stomach and the head for the full feeling.

Many people have learned to over-ride the ability to recognise and respond to the full, satisfied feeling. Unfortunately for many, this ability is de-activated very early in life as a baby or as a young toddler.

Babies are born with a natural mechanism that can tell when the stomach is full. When babies and toddlers feel full they push the breast, bottle or plate away. They refuse to eat more.

Many parents or caregivers will then insist the child eat more. Assuming with concern that, 'surely that wasn't enough, 'just a little more', or even, 'you must finish what was on the plate or in the bottle'.

The CPR audios address this issue often. They help you remember that it's okay to push the plate away and that it is even okay to leave food on the plate. When you tune in or check-in with your stomach between mouthfuls, you allow your brain and stomach to reactivate the full satisfied feeling again.

When you begin to do this, you'll notice you only need a third to a half of the quantity you have been served.

This commitment is definitely about giving you permission to slow down, tune in and listen. As soon as you feel comfortable or satisfied, simply commit to push the plate away.

Even making the movement with your hands to push your plate away as you repeat to yourself, 'enough is enough'. The CPR audios repeat this suggestion often. After a few days you might even begin to hear yourself echo 'Enough is enough, I push the plate away', as you check in between mouthfuls.

- After you swallow, pause and 'check in' or 'tune' into the stomach. Listen out for the comfortable, satisfied feeling or that inner knowing that 'enough is enough'.
- Put your knife and fork down between mouthfuls. If you are eating finger food or a sandwich, put the food down on the plate after each bite and pause as you 'check' in. This makes it easier for your brain to consciously tune in to the full feeling, and recognise when 'enough is enough'.
- It is important that you also do not eat in front of the television or while reading or working on the computer, or while driving. This will be explained in more detail in Chapter 8.

Have you ever snacked while watching a movie? Did you reach for more and the popcorn, chips or chocolate was finished? Your mind was focused on the movie, not on the snack. You were eating on automatic pilot.

That's what happens when you eat in front of the television or while busy with other things. You eat more than you really needed because there was minimal enjoyment, leading to less satisfaction, and less likelihood of recognising the full feeling.

Remember, the mind does not know the difference between real and imagined, so the mind needs to 'see' the food disappear from the plate so that it can trigger the satisfied, comfortable feeling.

**So the keys to this commitment are:**

- Look at the food disappearing from the plate
- Put your knife and fork, or sandwich down between bites
- Chew 15-30 times and then, swallow
- Pause to check-in to your stomach between mouthfuls, listen for the satisfied or comfortable feeling

- *Push the plate away* the moment you sense enough is enough
- You have permission to leave food on your plate

Once you are ready to read Chapter 8, pause between mouthfuls, check-in with your stomach for the satisfied feeling and push the plate away, please accept this commitment:

Signature:                                                          Date:

## COMMITMENT SIX

### Make Food Choices with your Stomach - not your mouth or head

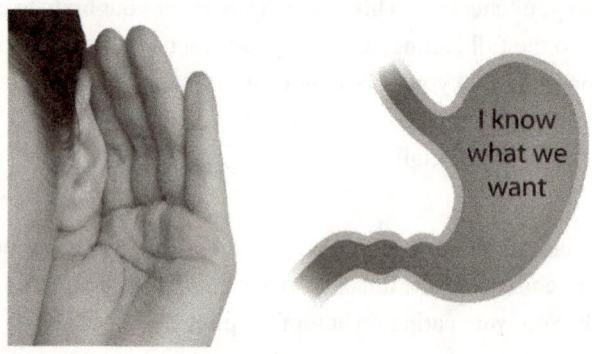

I know what we want

Many people with unhealthy eating habits, including *snacking, picking or grazing,* tend to eat unconsciously. If they are semi-conscious about it, they often do it anyway and berate themselves afterwards. *"I can't believe I finished that bar of chocolate or packet of chips".*

The trick to mastering this issue is to:

a) Use the CPR audios

b) Become more conscious of how you choose food, why, and when you choose it. The how and when will become easier the more you follow the commitments and listen to the audios. The 'Why' you choose certain foods, will become easier to control once you read Chapter 3 onwards.

The key to this commitment is: Choose food with your stomach not your head or your mouth.

If you or someone you know has developed habits associated with over indulging in sweets, savouries, snacking, picking and grazing; even addictions and habits to specific foods, then choosing food consciously with the stomach, rather than the head or mouth may seem challenging at first. If there is a habit or belief that generates thoughts like '*I have to have something sweet to finish off the meal',* then the same challenge may apply.

In the past, the decision about which food you choose, or if you need any food at all, was made by what the 'greedy eyes see', what the 'greedy mouth wants' or what the 'greedy appetite' in the head says.

If you consulted your stomach instead at this time, if you paused to 'check in' with your stomach to find out whether it was genuinely hungry and, if so, what nutrition it needed, I guarantee your stomach would reject the unhealthy choice, the sugary, starchy food or the snack.

Now, communicating with your stomach about which food you really want, or if you need any food at all, may seem like a strange thing to do. However, I guarantee that once you start consulting your stomach about food types and quantity, you will begin to choose healthier options more easily.

If your stomach were genuinely hungry, it would be happier to have a healthy protein, vegetable or fruit to satisfy its need for nutrition. It would feel uncomfortable if consulted about starchy carbohydrates, processed sugars or chemically enhanced science projects like processed foods.

Stomachs are not greedy; mouths, eyes and heads have been taught how to be greedy. Mouths, eyes and heads have learned to crave sugary, processed starchy chemically enhanced 'food'. Your stomach only ever wants nutritious life giving food.

When you consult your stomach about what it wants to eat, it will feel 'lighter' when nutritious foods are offered and heavier when starchy processed foods are presented. If you consulted your stomach every time you had the urge to pick, snack or graze between meals, your stomach would indicate whether you really needed nutrition, whether it was genuinely hungry, or if the 'hunger' was actually greedy appetite at play.

This issue is addressed with the CPR audios often. Throughout many of the audios there are specific suggestions to help you distinguish between genuine hunger and habitual or greedy cravings. The audios will help you differentiate between head and mouth hunger or the genuine need for nutrition.

I have also provided other techniques in Chapters 3 and 4 to help you program and rewire greedy appetite so that you can easily stop cravings.

In relation to this commitment however I simply ask that you start to interrupt the thought or craving by consulting your stomach first. Consult your stomach, 'tune-in' to sense if it needs anything at all.

Once you begin using the CPR audios to help disengage head, eye and mouth hunger, this will become even easier to do.

Remember, this does not mean you will never eat another sweet, chocolate, pastry, cake, potato crisp or chip, bread or unhealthy snack again. It simply means you will want them less often, and, you will be satisfied with less of them. There are no banned foods when you unzip the fat suit.

So Commitment Six is simply: Make your decision about which food, or whether you are hungry at all, from your stomach, instead of your mouth, eyes or head.

**Consult your stomach and ask:**

*How will my stomach feel a half hour after eating this (name of food)?*

*Is my stomach genuinely hungry or is it my head or mouth that wants this (name of food)?*

If the foods you consulted your stomach about were starchy, sugary, processed or unhealthy, the feeling would be uncomfortable. The stomach needs nutritious food for the body to live. The stomach is not greedy, it will feel good (lighter) when you consult it about nutritious food, and it will feel heavy, sluggish and uncomfortable, if you consult it about greedy appetite food.

**Once you are ready to commit to consult or check-in with your stomach more often before choosing food, and to read about how to conquer greedy appetite and unhelpful cravings in Chapters 3 and 4, then please accept this commitment:**

**Signature:**                                          **Date:**

## COMMITMENT SEVEN

### Serve Smaller Portions

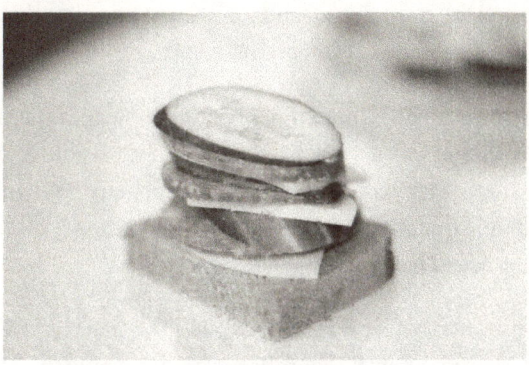

This commitment is self-explanatory. Make the commitment to yourself to serve smaller amounts of food, on a smaller plate.

In our fast food society where *'super size me'* or *'would you like to add fries with that?',* and where cooking shows and fancy presentation of food have become fashionable, we have seen the growth of the humble dinner plate. Plates and food portions have become fashionably huge! Our greedy appetite, mouth, eye and head hunger have been trained to want more. The old saying that the 'eyes are bigger than the belly' could not be any truer today.

It's time to recognise the difference between what is a healthy portion and what has become 'normal'. Healthy is a small meal with a protein base and healthy vegetables or salad as the side. Today's 'normal' has become supersized and abnormal.

I consulted with a client who lost 28 kilograms and reached a plateau. She couldn't seem to shift any more weight, but was still 14 kilograms away from her goal.

I assessed her exercise routine; and together we worked on emotional issues and past patterns. Each time I would ask her about her portion size. She assured me her meals were on the smaller side of normal. Still she did not move towards her goal. One day, I had an appointment with her at around lunchtime. She brought her lunch with her to the clinic; it was a very healthy chicken salad.

The choice was wonderful, healthy, fresh, and nutritious with protein, salad and vegetables. The size of the meal however, could have fed two people. On another occasion she showed me the portion size of a soup that her husband had made.

Once again the portion was double what the stomach really needed. As her husband is a chef, the large portion size had become normal to her. These portions had become the 'normal size' the family ate for every meal.

She promptly adjusted the portion size and the weight began to shift again. By the next week she had lost another 1.2 kilograms.

**Assess what is normal to you**. Contemplate your stomach as the size of your fist (approximately). If you chewed your food into a paste would it fit *comfortably* inside that stomach (fist) or would it stretch its capacity? When the food you choose is balanced nutritionally, you only need as much food, when chewed, that would fit inside your fist. That is normal.

So gradually begin to downsize, don't supersize. The capacity of your stomach will shrink within days, and you'll feel fuller faster very quickly. The CPR audios will help you do this by reinforcing *'smaller portions, healthy options, it's the easiest thing I've ever done'*.

**Smaller Portion Tips:**

- Choose protein first (meat, chicken, fish etc) approximately 50-70 grams of protein per meal
- Include a protein with every meal including breakfast
- Select your vegetables or salad to accompany the protein
- Invest in smaller bowls and plates. Choose special/attractive crockery that entices you to use it
- Discover what is normal - assess the size of your fist
- Pause before eating compare what is on your plate with what would fit inside your fist once it was chewed to a paste.
- Check in to see what portion size a slim and healthy person eats and compare it to how much you have served yourself
- Use one of the exercises in Chapter 4 or the Control audio to dissolve cravings if you suspect that greedy appetite wants more on the plate than you need
- Remember you can leave food and push the plate away

Once you feel ready to commit to re-discover what 'normal' portion sizes are, serve less and use smaller crockery, then please accept this commitment:

**Signature:**                                                      **Date:**

## COMMITMENT EIGHT

### Rewire for Hydration – Thirsty for water

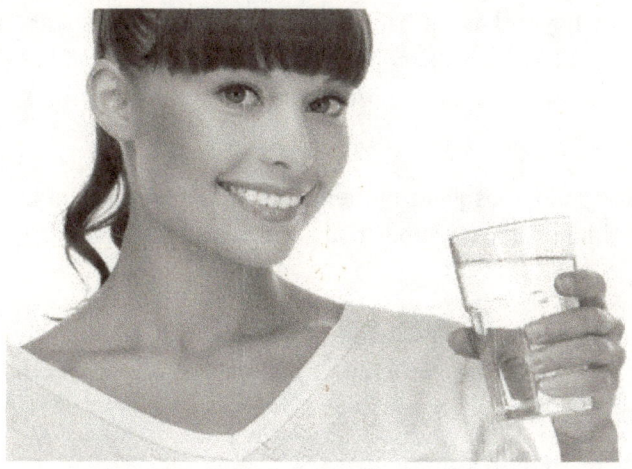

People reduce weight simply by drinking more water. You've heard it all before, drink at least 6-8 glasses or 2 litres of water every day. I agree with this completely, however I will clarify why.

**Importance of water for the mind and body:**

Your brain is 75% water. Your memory, your thinking, your chemical reactions in your brain and body and your emotional and hormonal states, rely upon how hydrated your brain is.

Many headaches can be solved by drinking water because a headache is one of the main signs of dehydration.

- Water helps to regulate your body temperature
- It carry nutrients and oxygen to the cells of your body
- Water moistens the oxygen so breathing is easier
- Your blood needs water. It is made up of about 83% water
- Water accounts for 22 % of your bones
- It cushions your joints. It protects the joints and bones from damage
- You need water to convert food to energy. It helps you absorb nutrients
- It helps protect and cushion your organs
- Your muscles rely on water. It accounts for up 75% of muscle content
- It helps you eliminate waste from your body

Some people assume that their daily intake of 6-8 glasses of liquid can include fizzy sugary drinks, alcohol and caffeine based drinks. Although these contain some water, *they cannot be used by the body as water*. These drinks add toxins to the body and the body then needs more water to eliminate and process those sugars and toxins. If you have a habit associated with fizzy, sugary drinks, alcohol or caffeine, please use the craving control techniques and the Control audios to eliminate these cravings. Ensure you drink at least 2 litres of *pure water* each day.

I also recommend adding a squeeze of lemon or lime first thing in the morning to water; this helps alkalise your body and stimulates digestion and the metabolism.

**Remember drinking pure water is vital to our survival. We can live much longer without food than we can without water.** *(I don't recommend trying either by the way)*

**Drinking water at certain times maximises its effectiveness too:**

2 glasses of water after waking - helps activate internal organs

1 glass of water 30 minutes before a meal – helps digestion

1 glass of water before taking a bath – helps lower blood pressure

1 glass of water before going to bed – helps avoids stroke or heart attack

According to medical experts: water before bedtime also helps to prevent leg cramps

So are you getting the picture ….? Pitcher of water that is?

**Once you consciously choose to increase your water intake to a healthy level (if you don't already do so), then please accept this commitment:**

**Signature:**                                               **Date:**

## COMMITMENT NINE

### Choose to Wiggle It - Rewire Healthy Movement of the Body

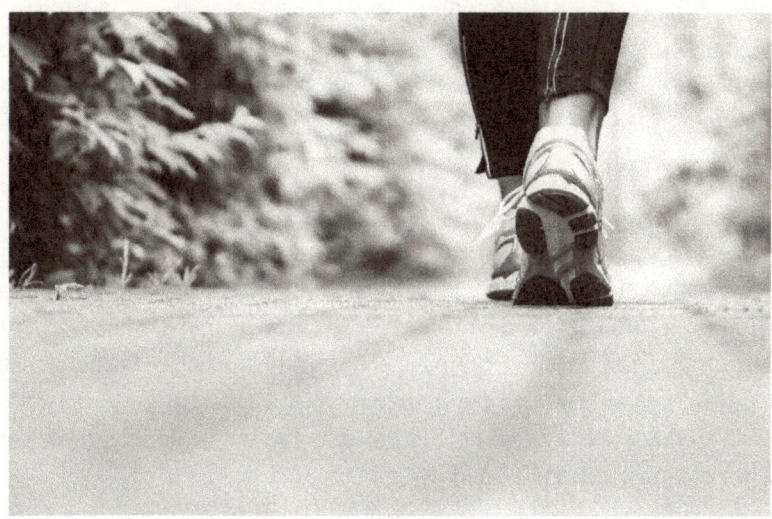

The 'exercise' issue challenges many people. Some people are naturally motivated to move their body; others find it a chore, but grudgingly do it anyway. Others create excuses to avoid it at all costs and prioritise life without it.

**Completing this commitment daily is vital so that you can reduce excess fat and gain overall physical health and stamina. This topic is so important that I have devoted the whole of Chapter 9 to this subject. I have also provided a *Program Audio* called *Motivation to Move My Body & Exercise* and two versions of a Rewire audio to stimulate healthy movement every day.**

As I have devoted a whole chapter and *Program and Rewire* audios to help you fulfil this commitment, I will not say much more about this topic here other than:

Twenty to thirty minutes a day of appropriate movement is all it takes. (If your fitness level or general health requires medical attention, please consult your health care practitioner before starting a physical fitness program).

**If you do not move your body daily (appropriate to your level of fitness and health), your body will metabolise unused muscle. You will lose muscle mass and strength, rather than burn off excess fat and kilos.**

Movement communicates to your body that you want to use your muscles. It will therefore burn excess kilos and fat instead of muscle mass and strength.

Walk, skip, and dance even if it's around the house. Forget the word 'exercise', simply *choose to move* and make it fun! Indulge in 'incidental' movement. Do the housework or wash the car more vigorously. Park further away from work or the shopping centre. Take a few trips to the washing line instead of only one to hang out the washing. Find ways to work up a healthy sweat in your everyday life, and you will be burning off the excess much faster.

It really doesn't matter *what movement* you do; simply *move more*.

I had a very unfit and obese client who was embarrassed about going out in public to exercise; even walking was not an option due to the pain in her knees from her excess size. Once she changed her perspective from 'exercise' to 'movement', she started walking laps around the lounge room. Listening to the *Program and Rewire* audios made it easier as she continued, but in the beginning, these small steps kept her injury free and started the process of change.

If you have diabetes or a medical condition, then please consult your healthcare practitioner and monitor your blood sugar levels carefully. As you begin to unzip the extra kilos and get fitter, your medical practitioner may need to discuss or adjust medication for you. So if you do have these health issues, please inform your GP of your intent to unzip the fat suit and move your body more!

**Once you feel ready to commit to read Chapter 9, and use the 'Motivation to Move My Body & Exercise' audio, then please accept this commitment:**

**Signature:**                                                    **Date:**

## COMMITMENT TEN

### Feed the Mind – Your Progress Journal to Success

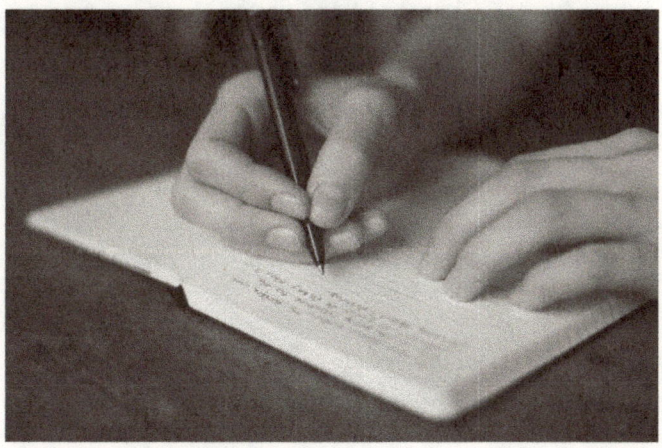

This commitment takes us back to two of my original Keys

**1: Real or imagined -** 'The mind doesn't know the difference between real and imagined, what the mind sees it believes.'

**2: Imagination** – Mind Rehearsal. The method by which the brain can learn better habits, thoughts and feelings.

Chapter 14 is dedicated to this commitment and I have provided your Progress Journal there. This is no ordinary journal. The progress journal in Chapter 14 has been adapted from a wonderful technique called 'The Dear Diary Process' which was devised by a highly respected colleague (Stuart Walter). Stuart specialises in the psychology of success in the sporting arena. He works with top athletes to help them achieve higher standards in their chosen field. The journaling technique takes advantage of the fact that your brain does not know the difference between real and imagined. It encourages you to use mind rehearsal to create new ' maps' or blueprints for how you will think and behave as you move toward your slim and healthy outcomes.

So Chapter 14 helps you focus in a very specific way on your goals for your body. I have adapted Stuart's 'Dear Diary Process' with his permission and provided your *'Progress Journal for Success'*. This will support you to unzip the fat suit and think slim and healthy even faster.

For now, all I ask is that you be aware that one of your commitments will be to write or draw or imagine your successful outcomes are here already. All will be explained in detail in Chapter 14.

**Once you commit to read Chapter 14 and accept that Commitment 10 asks you to use mind rehearsal in a particular way when you get there, then please accept this commitment:**

**Signature:**                                                          **Date:**

| | The 10 commitments | Commitments Summary |
|---|---|---|
| 1 | Map your Progress – Mind Rehearse wearing goal outfit in your new size | Rehearse Outfit |
| 2 | Listen to at least one CPR audio daily from the Unzip the Fat Suit Program | Audio Daily |
| 3 | Weigh in once per week | Weigh Once |
| 4 | Rewire digestion - Choose to chew slowly | Chew Slowly |
| 5 | Push the plate away as soon as you feel comfortable. *'Check in' to your stomach between mouthfuls for the satisfied feeling* | Push Plate |
| 6 | Make food choices with your stomach not your mouth or head. *'Check in' with your stomach before choosing food for what feels light/healthy* | Stomach chooses |
| 7 | Serve smaller portions – on a smaller plate | Smaller Portions |
| 8 | Rewire for hydration – thirsty for water | Thirst = Water |
| 9 | Choose to wiggle it – move your body more | Wiggle Move |
| 10 | Feed your mind – progress journal to success | Write Progress |

**If you haven't already downloaded a COMMITMENT REMINDER CHART or summary table do so now.**

| Remember your 10 Commitments |
|:---:|
| Rehearse Outfit |
| Audio Daily |
| Weigh Once |
| Stomach Chooses |
| Smaller Portions |
| Chew Slowly |
| Push Plate |
| Thirst = Water |
| Wiggle Move |
| Write Progress |

Feel free to download as many times as you wish. Laminate the reminder chart or summary table. Put them around the house to help remind you of your commitments daily. Put one inside the pantry or on the fridge, or on the bathroom mirror. Anywhere that helps remind you to check in with your plan.

People who complete the 10 Commitments daily - Unzip the fat suit more easily and permanently.

# THREE

---

## Control & Conquer Greedy Appetite

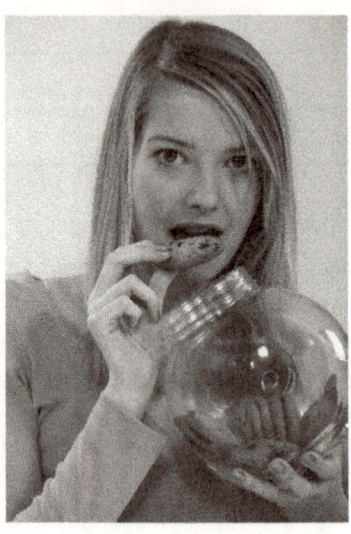

The purpose of this chapter is to introduce four very important strategies to help you unzip the fat suit permanently.

By reading and using the strategies and questionnaires in this chapter you will be able to:

1. Recognise and understand the different types of Hunger including

   a. Genuine
   b. Emotional
   c. Stress
   d. Habitual
   e. Boredom
   f. Comfort

2. Respond appropriately to genuine hunger
3. Respond appropriately to unhelpful hungers
4. Control and eliminate unhelpful 'hungers' with the strategies provided

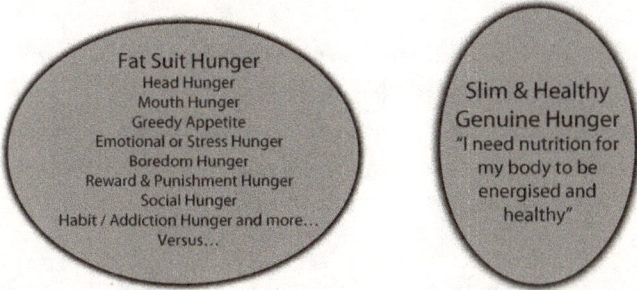

In this chapter I have also provided two helpful questionnaires. These questionnaires help you ascertain why you are more likely to crave or eat certain foods at certain times, and what (if any) your unhelpful attachments to food might be. This information will help you discover the types of appropriate or inappropriate hungers that have kept you in the fat suit for too long.

In order to unzip the fat suit permanently, you need to understand your relationship with food and eating. The first questionnaire will help you determine the types of foods and triggers that are unhelpful to you.

Later in the chapter, the second questionnaire called the ***Greedy Appetite 'Why Questionnaire',*** provides a way to cross check these challenges from a slightly different perspective. This will help you become aware of the patterns that trigger fat suit cravings and unhelpful hungers.

Both questionnaires help you recognise your different types of hungers and cravings and the triggers that cause them. Once you have a clearer picture of the times, people, events or circumstances that trigger greedy appetite or 'fat suit' eating, then you can begin to use the CPR audios, and other techniques in the book, to control and conquer your reactions, before they cause you to eat.

When you recognise the different types of hungers specific to different triggers, such as boredom or stress hungers, social or comfort hungers, habitual and even rebellion hunger too, then you can learn how to control the cravings associated with them. Once you have listened to the *Control audios* and the other *Program and Rewire* audios enough, you will automatically begin to make better choices for your body permanently.

**Do you understand the relationship you have to different types of foods in different circumstances? Are you aware of the types of food you are triggered to eat in response to the types of hunger you experience?**

For example:

- Do you look specifically for chocolate when you're stressed
- Is bread the thing that satisfies you when you're bored
- Are biscuits, cakes and sweets what you want when you're hurt /upset
- To finish off a meal, are savoury and salty snacks satisfying, or is something sweet required

Once you understand the links that are specific to you and you use the techniques and *Control audios* provided in this chapter, then you can begin to disengage those links. (You simply won't react in that unhelpful way anymore).

You can then easily choose to do something more appropriate until those reactions have been eliminated permanently.

Examples of these possible links might be:

- Emotional Upset = comfort hunger = *"Where's the chocolate"*
- Coffee with friends = social hunger = *"Her muffin looks nice, I'll have one too"*
- Argument = rebellion/punishment hunger = *"Give me the whole pack, I'll show you!"*
- Home alone = boredom/comfort hunger = *"What's in the pantry?"*

Take a few moments to think about the types of hungers in the first questionnaire. Assess whether or not they apply to you. Some will and some won't. Respond only to the ones that relate to you. It's for your eyes only, so be as honest as you can. Doing this will help you overcome inappropriate eating patterns.

Think about the types of triggers that may have stimulated those hungers in the past too. Consider the different types of foods you usually choose to satisfy the hunger. Write everything down that comes to you as you consider each hunger type; perhaps you might be able to 'hear' your automatic response, or you might become aware of a feeling or sensation in your body or mouth.

| Unhelpful Hunger Questionnaire | | | |
|---|---|---|---|
| **Types of Unhelpful Hunger** | **What are the Common triggers that stimulate this type of hunger?** | **Which foods do you choose to satisfy it?** For example: sweet, savoury or a specific food if you are aware of it | **Is there anything else you recall?** Any thoughts, emotions, body sensations? |
| **Greedy Appetite** Do you eat just because it's there, or even if you are already full and then wish you hadn't? (Eyes bigger than your belly). | | | |
| **Reward Hunger** Do you use food as a reward/ perhaps at the completion of a task or when you have done well? | | | |
| **Social Hunger** Is food a part of your social life, do you eat more when with friends even if you are not hungry? Do you find it hard to say no if others are eating? | | | |
| **Comfort Hunger** Do you use food to comfort you when you feel sorry for yourself or hurt or in pain? | | | |
| **Boredom Hunger** Do you eat if you are bored or lonely? | | | |
| **Stress Hunger** Do you eat in times of high stress? Do you use food to calm or give you more energy to deal with stress? Do you 'chew' on food while you think about how to handle the stressful situation? | | | |

*(continued)*

| Type of Hunger | Common triggers | Which food you reach for? | Anything else to share? |
|---|---|---|---|
| **Control / Rebellion Hunger** Do you eat when you are angry or resentful or when someone says you shouldn't? Or if you feel threatened or out of control in some way? | | | |
| **Habitual / addiction Hunger** Do you physically crave foods at certain times of the day and does your body respond with physical symptoms if you don't eat it? | | | |
| **Head Hunger (thoughts about food)** Do you have constant repetitive thoughts about certain foods at certain times? Do you obsess about eating even when you are not genuinely hungry? | | | |
| **Mouth Hunger (craving for food)** Do you experience strong sensations/ cravings in your mouth when you think about or want certain foods? | | | |
| **Punishment / Sabotage Hunger** Do you use food to punish yourself if you make a mistake? Or if you are doing well at weight reduction or if someone compliments you? | | | |
| **Exhaustion Hunger** Do you grab whatever food you can when you are tired, it doesn't matter what? Or when you think you deserve a pick me up? | | | |
| **Other** For any other reason? | | | |

Whether you choose to fill this questionnaire out now or as you go through the book, your responses will help you use the control cravings techniques in the next chapter. Your responses will help you recognise which unhelpful habits and triggers are connected to which foods, so you can disconnect the links that are not helping you.

If you haven't already begun to use the *Control audios* then start today. In Chapter 4 I explain what the Control tapping technique is and how it works. You will also learn how to use the Control tapping techniques without the audios too. For now use the control audios and simply follow along with what I say word for word. If you prefer you can also watch one of the demonstration control craving video tutorials on my YouTube channel. http://www.youtube.com/MaggieWilde

Before you get to Chapter 4 however, there are a number of other very useful techniques you can use to begin taking control of your eating triggers and specific food habits.

You can begin rewiring your habits immediately with this assessment technique by Dr Caroline Leaf. Dr Leaf is a leading Brain and Learning Specialist who has spent years researching the human brain. Her research focuses on how to unlock the brain's potential and how negative thinking affects it. Dr Leaf suggests some great strategies to detox the mind from unhelpful thoughts. I have adapted one of her techniques to relate specifically to food and eating to help you break the cycle of greedy appetite and unhelpful emotional eating habits.

In her book *"Who Switched off My Brain? Controlling toxic thoughts and emotions,"* Dr Leaf explains how thoughts are created in the brain and how important it is to distinguish between helpful thoughts, and unhelpful ones. She calls it 'Detoxing your brain'.

Dr Leaf believes that approximately 15% to 35% of what you read, what you see and hear is important and stored in the brain as memory. She also suggests that to have a healthy mind and body, we should detox 65% to 85% of the rest of the information. She says it's "superfluous".

Her research consistently reveals that when we haven't understood or can't deal with all this excess information, then our brain becomes overwhelmed and creates toxic thoughts. It's like a child that eats too much sugar; it starts behaving in silly ways! Our brain does the same thing when it 'eats' too much superfluous information; it becomes overloaded and shuts down. It starts to 'think' in silly ways.

Dr Leaf suggests *"in order to build strong neural connections, strong memory and healthier thoughts about yourself and your body, you need to approach all information coming into your brain with a filter."* She calls it a '*strainer*'.

77

Dr Leaf's 'strainer' is a simple strategy she calls:

**"Ask-answer-discuss"**

By having an internal 'ask-answer-discuss' chat, you begin to select the 15-35% of information that you do need to build a strong healthy mind and memory, and then discard or reject the rest as irrelevant. It helps you reframe or approach your thoughts; actions and emotions from a more helpful perspective.

### *Unzip the fat suit example:*

If you have tried 5 plus different diets and read lots of articles or books on food, your brain can become overwhelmed with information about what to do to lose weight. One book tells you fats are bad, another says you should only eat protein and others say cabbage is the 'cure'. So many do's and don't's, should's and shouldn'ts, no wonder we become overwhelmed.

According to Dr Leaf, this conflicting information can create a build up of confusion that leads to toxic thoughts and 'helpless' feelings.

From my professional standpoint, I believe this overload and confusion creates procrastination and stagnancy. No matter how many times you make the commitment to achieve your goal, you lose focus and simply give up. This leads to self-recrimination and disappointment. It becomes a vicious cycle and creates the yo-yo dieter who can't get off the merry-go-round.

My suggestion is to use Dr Leafs 'strainer' theory to help you understand the triggers that cause subconscious cravings and unhelpful emotions, inappropriate hungers and toxic thinking. When cravings or greedy appetite hungers occur, you can **'Ask-answer-discuss'** by holding an internal question and answer time. The list of example questions below, provide a sample of how I use this method successfully with clients. The questions in this list can be adapted to suit you:

If you are triggered to crave food by a specific event, emotion or person, ask internally:

- Is this reaction / craving / hunger moving me towards my goal or away from it?
- What triggered this reaction or craving?
- What am I trying to achieve by craving this food? (For example: comfort, confidence, something to do)
- Is there something more helpful I could do now, that would satisfy my need for…(comfort or other need) and move me toward my goal?

What could I do to respond differently right now?

You don't need to have all the answers now, but by holding an internal discussion, it's like turning a light switch on in a dark room. Suddenly you can see what you couldn't see before. You will bring subconscious habits out of darkness (out of your control) into light (into your control). You are then more likely to interrupt the subconscious mind's old unhelpful dark instinct to *'reach for the carbohydrate or comfort food'* and make a 'lighter' or healthier choice.

By pausing to do this, it gives your mind time to consider and reject the old unhelpful pattern. When you practice this often, the choice becomes easier each time. You don't have to be perfect; simply aim to be better at it today, than you were yesterday.

According to Dr Leaf, internal discussions like this develop deeper more helpful neural connections. She says, *"Correct, positive thinking is also shown in research to 'grow' your brain. Toxic thoughts also grow your brain, but not in beneficial ways."* Dr Leaf adds, *"They will weigh down your whole body, mind and spirit."*

Notice the use of the words 'weigh down'? It is not simply the cravings that are weighing you down, but also the toxic thoughts and emotions that are created as a result of reacting to the cravings. *"I wish I hadn't done that"*. Or *"I can't believe I did that again"* or *"See I'm useless, hopeless"*.

It is important to note that by using the internal discussion strategy, you are creating newer, more positive thinking patterns. You can literally change the cravings by shining a light on them and internally discussing alternatives. The brain rewires new connections over the old ones. You begin to respond more consciously around food and old triggers.

According to Dr Leaf's research, you must never let cravings, desires or unhelpful thoughts about food travel through your mind unchecked. If this occurs you will eventually reach that point where you don't have control over the impulses or the triggers that cause them.

In other words those thoughts will become automatic and habitual.

The following questionnaire will address the types of greedy appetite and unhelpful hungers that might be running unchecked in your brain. By completing this second questionnaire, you can cross check to ensure you shine as much light as you can on unhelpful eating patterns and food associations. This way you can have more ammunition to help you reinforce new helpful connections.

# The Greedy Appetite 'Why Questionnaire'

(This test and scorecard has been adapted to help you unzip the fat suit for good by Maggie Wilde from an original concept by the American Academy of Family Physicians to help establish the motivation for habits like smoking. As the habitual process of hand to mouth feeding can be similar to that of using cigarettes or any other oral substance, the adaptation of this questionnaire is helpful to shine a light on any subconscious gains for poor eating habits).

Next to the following statements, mark the number that best describes your own experience with regard to greedy, poor, lazy, unhealthy or overeating habits …

5 = Always
4 = Most of the time
3 = Once in a while
2 = Rarely
1 = Never


\_\_\_\_ A. I eat to boost my energy

\_\_\_\_ B. Handling/preparing food is part of the enjoyment of eating it

\_\_\_\_ C. Eating is pleasant and relaxing

\_\_\_\_ D. I eat when I feel angry

\_\_\_\_ E. When I am out of my favourite 'binge' foods, I think about them until I can get more

\_\_\_\_ F. I eat automatically, without being aware of it sometimes

\_\_\_\_ G. I always eat bad/fat suit/unhelpful foods when people around me are eating them

\_\_\_\_ H. I eat to make me feel better, to perk myself up

\_\_\_\_ I. Part of my enjoyment from eating is the preparation of food

\_\_\_\_ J. I get pleasure from eating bad/fat suit/unhelpful foods

\_\_\_\_ K. When I feel uncomfortable or upset, I eat

\_\_\_\_ L. When I'm not eating food, I'm very much aware that I am thinking of food

\_\_\_\_ M. I often reach for more when I'm still chewing

\_\_\_\_ N. I eat with friends when I am having a good time

_____ O. When I eat, part of the enjoyment is watching the food disappear

_____ P. I want food most often when I am comfortable and relaxed

_____ Q. I eat when I am "unhappy" or "feeling down" and want to take my mind off what bothers me

_____ R. I get hunger pangs in between meals

_____ S. I've found myself chewing food and haven't consciously remembered eating it

_____ T. I always think about what to eat when I am socialising with friends at a party or bar

_____ U. I always eat to get a lift in my mood

## Now Score Yourself

**Step 1:** Transfer the numbers you marked on the quiz to the scorecard by matching up the letters. For example, take the number you wrote for question A on the Questionnaire and enter it on line A of the scorecard.

**Step 2:** Add each set of 3 scores on the scorecard to get the total for each different category. For example, to find your score on the "It stimulates me" category, add together the scores for questions A, H and U.

The score for each category can range from a low of 3 to a high of 15. A score of 11 or above on any set is high and means that your eating is probably influenced by that category. A score of 7 or below is low and means that this category is not a primary source of satisfaction to you when you eat.

Refer to the following scorecard to discover the results.

### Greedy Appetite 'Why' Test Score Card

**"It stimulates me."** You feel that overeating gives you energy and keeps you going. Think about alternative ways to boost your energy. A brisk walk or using the strategies from the book and Control audios will help. Also use the head hunger interruptions discussed in Chapter 4 or any other CPR audio from the program.

_____ A   _____ H   _____ U   _____ "Stimulation, eating that food gives me energy"
     **Total**

**"I want something to do."** There are a lot of things you can do to fill in your time without eating. Use the suggestions for craving control and pattern interruptions in Chapter 4. Use the Control audios or the tapping exercises outlined in the next chapter too. Start a healthy hobby, take up yoga or read something motivational.

___ B ___ I ___ O ___ "It's about boredom, having something to do"
**Total**

**"It feels good."** You get a lot of physical and emotional pleasure from eating. Various forms of movement or any of the CPR audios can be effective alternatives because they stimulate positive endorphins in the brain. These create natural 'feel good' highs and they are natural pain-killers and positive emotion stimulators.

___ C ___ J ___ P            ___ "Pleasure/Relaxation Eater"
**Total**

**"It's a crutch."** If you find foods comforting in times of stress this book and the CPR audios are exactly what you need. I have provided many techniques and audios so that you can deal with and reduce stress in more helpful ways. Check out Chapter 12 and use the Be Stress Free Program audio.

___ D ___ K ___ Q            ___ "Crutch/Tension/Stress Eater"
**Total**

**"I'm hooked."** In addition to perhaps having a psychological addiction to excess or unhealthy foods, you may also have a physical reliance on the sugars or salts. It is important to be aware that within a short time of reducing your intake of unhealthy, high sugar/fat and/or salty foods, you will stop craving these types of foods. Use techniques such as Control audios to dissolve cravings. Use other strategies such as tapping in Chapter 4 or Dr Leaf's 'Strainer' technique from this chapter. These will help break the addiction. You will be back in control of your eating habits sooner than you think. Use other CPR audios such as the Control cravings audio or the Rewire audios, the demonstration videos or Eliminate Greedy Appetite Program audio.

___ E ___ L ___ R            ___ "I'm addicted ... Craving/Addiction"
**Total**

**"It's part of my routine."** If unhealthy food choices are merely part of your routine, stopping should be relatively easy. Become aware of every morsel and why or what stimulated you to put it in your mouth. Keep a progress journal, it will be a good way to do this. (Refer to Chapter 14). Also go back to your 'Why'. Focusing on your most important reasons for being slim and healthy will motivate you to 'break' the routine. Use Dr Leaf's 'ask, answer and discuss' strategy to shine light on the habit in your conscious mind. You'll soon realise how easy it is to be back in control of choosing how you use your time and treat your body.

___ F  ___ M  ___ S                                              ___ "It's a habit"
    **Total**

**"Food is a social thing for me."** You eat when people around you are eating even if you are not hungry. You eat when someone offers you something whether you are hungry or not. It is important for you to feel more confident about being in control of your food choices. Use the CPR audios and strategies from the previous paragraph to dissolve the urges. Focus on the Control audios and the Rewire Self Confidence audio. If you cannot avoid a social situation associated with food then choose smaller portions and the healthiest option. Remember my comments about '*instant gratification syndrome*'? It's not about 'I can't have it ever again'. It's about maybe I'll have it another time, less of it and less often.

___ G  ___ N  ___ T
___ "The Social Eater" says; '*Oh what the heck....Just this once won't hurt*'
    **Total**

Once you know your unhelpful eating patterns and the types of hungers you respond to, you can begin to recognise the warning signs. When you recognise these warning signs, you can use any or all of the strategies I have discussed so far to interrupt the pattern of the past. Try the internal discussion I outlined and/or use the Control and Rewire audios to start with. There are lots of other strategies in the following chapters too. Start practicing the tapping exercises in Chapter 4. These will help make it easier to stay on track.

## Other Helpful Strategies

Remember: Head, mouth, boredom or emotional hunger, stress or habitual hunger refer to a state whereby you *think* or *feel* that you need or want food, but your body is not actually the one that is in need of energy. Your mind is stimulating thoughts that create sensations in your body or mouth. Those thoughts and sensations cause the urge to eat.

**The only true reason for anyone to eat - is to provide nutrition for the body to live.**

Our love affair with food for pleasure, pain and power started as long ago as 500BC. Way back then, India discovered that you could extract natural cane juice to make edible sugar. Centuries later, we now use food for entertainment; we use it for comfort when we feel down, or to fill in time when we are bored. We use it to avoid, deny, punish or reward ourselves in a variety of different ways. We have used it as a power symbol; the rich could afford sugar, chocolate, coffee and spices, the poor filled their stomachs with bread and ate potatoes. In western cultures, eating to provide nutrition for the body, took a back seat to eating for pleasure, pain and power a long time ago. No wonder we have such ingrained subconscious emotional confusion about food.

So from today, every time you think you are hungry, it is important to assess whether the trigger for food is a genuine need for nutrition or an emotional subconscious pattern (map), masquerading as genuine hunger. (Remember Granny's comfort cuddle/biscuit?)

If choosing the unhealthy option or snacking in between meals is simply a habitual response and has no emotional attachment or physical addiction, then using a conscious mind strategy like an internal discussion, will be helpful to shine light on the habit and stop it. To do this, you can use the internal *ask, answer discuss questions* I outlined earlier in the chapter.

If there is a subconscious emotional pattern (such as granny's biscuit), or a physical addiction to the sugar or salt, then often no matter how much your conscious mind tries to switch off the craving, your subconscious will continue to stimulate it.

## Short Term Solution to Subconscious Emotional Eating Pattern or Addiction

If this is the case, you will at first need to use the *Control audios* in the short term to interrupt the craving or habit every time it happens. This will disconnect the link between the trigger that caused the craving, and the intensity of the desire to fulfil it will be eliminated.

## Long Term Solution to Subconscious Emotional Eating Pattern or Addiction

Continue to use the *Program and Rewire* audios daily. Once you have used the *Program and Rewire* audios often enough, then you won't need the *Control audios* at all. The link between the trigger for food and the subconscious emotional pattern or physical addiction, will have been disconnected.

No more programmed response to Granny's cuddle/biscuit.

Until this disconnection is permanent, you will need strategies to help determine which type of hunger it is before you respond to it. So do at least three things from my **'The Power of Three'** list.

By doing at least three of the strategies from this list you will interrupt the craving to eat the unhelpful/unhealthy food. The more you use the suggestions from this list, the easier the disconnection will be and the quicker you will gain control of your eating and be able to make healthier choices for your body.

If however, the desire for food was stimulated by genuine hunger, a genuine need for nutrition, then after doing *at least* three things from this list, you will recognise which type of hunger it is and be able to respond in a healthy way.

## The Power of Three

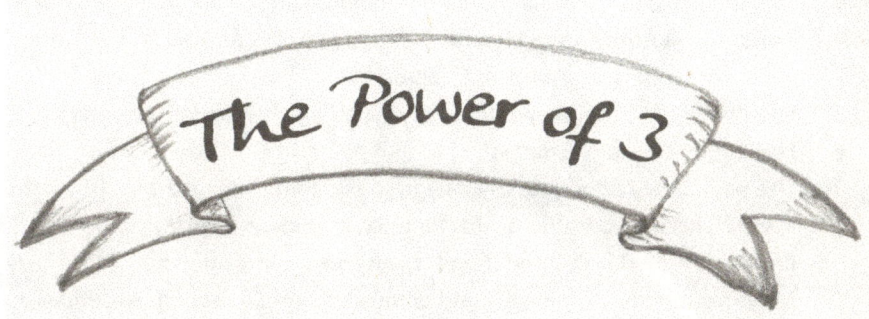

- Easy Solutions to Interrupt:
- Greedy Appetite
- Head and Mouth Cravings

## All other Emotional Hungers

If you suspect greedy appetite, head hunger, mouth hunger or some other emotional, subconscious stress 'hunger' is tricking you into thinking you are hungry, then simply commit to do **at least three** of these steps. Even if you are not sure whether the urge to eat is genuine hunger or an emotional or habitual craving, do at least 3 strategies, and you will be able to recognise the difference and respond appropriately.

When you follow this plan, you will feel more in control. You will always be able to interrupt and stop fat suit, greedy appetite hungers.

## Do at least three of *'The Power of Three'* techniques.

1. Drink 2 glasses of warm or room temperature water slowly (add a squeeze of lemon or lime if you like).
2. Concentrate on deep, slow belly breathing. Place your palm on your lower abdomen. Breathe in sending air down into your diaphragm. Genuine belly breaths cause the abdomen to expand (your belly will expand). Shallow breathing only causes the chest to rise. Deep belly breaths fill the diaphragm with air first and then the air expands up into the chest. (Do at least 6 deep belly breaths).
3. Acknowledge that the feeling will pass. Experience it with amusement and use a Control audio or tap on the karate point (refer to Chapter 4 for this technique) and say, *"I am in control, enough is enough"*.
4. Acknowledge the craving, desire or thought, and use the 'Ask - answer - discuss' questions from chapter 3. (To help with this, use the Control audios or tapping exercises in Chapter 4).
5. Use one of the Program audios (Eliminate Greedy Appetite or other).
6. Use a Rewire audio (Unzip the Fat Suit or Build Confidence).
7. Use one of the techniques to manage stress from Chapter 12.
8. Mind Rehearse your goal outfit. Imagine or pretend wearing it as if it fits already. Feel how good it feels 'as if' it's too big already.
9. Move your body with energy and enthusiasm for 60 seconds to stimulate "feel good" endorphins. For example repeatedly stand up and sit down, dance wiggle and move, stretch, do a yoga pose, while repeating silently in your mind "enough is enough".
10. Think about your most important reasons for being slim and healthy. Pretend in your mind as if it's already real. Write about it in your progress journal (see Chapter 14).

Read your 10 Commitments. Do one or more of them now. Consider the commitment you made to yourself when you signed them. Acknowledge that it's time to take responsibility.

- If you still feel hungry after doing at least three or more of these suggestions, it will be genuine hunger so...
- Eat a small nutritious snack such as nuts and seeds or a few grapes, (cup your hand and only eat an amount that fits into the palm)
- Eat each morsel one at a time, chew slowly and consciously. This helps your brain register that your body received nutrition. Be aware of each mouthful as you bring the snack to your mouth. Observe it disappear from your palm, be aware of the textures and flavours and eat it with joy. (Refer to Chapter 8)

## Give Yourself Support

It is important to recognise that as you experience changes that occur as a result of using the CPR audios and the 10 Commitments, you will frequently need to support yourself to continue. To do so requires that you *take ownership* of your plan and your goal. Focus on your 'Why's', take responsibility for and pride in what you are achieving and revel in each mini achievement along the way.

- Offer yourself positive inner encouragement. Use what I call your 'inner coach' instead of your 'inner critic'. (I'll discuss this further in Chapter 4)
- Reward yourself for the goals achieved when you reach a new milestone. It could be a massage or a facial, a manicure, a ticket to a game or whatever gives you joy
- Make a list of all your good points and achievements. Add to it and read it often to help you refocus
- Think of all the things, people or experiences you have to be grateful for
- Be kind to you, read your good points and achievements daily

Be compassionate to you, you may not be perfect, none of us are, but you are committed to be better than you were yesterday

**Print a free *'The Power of List'* and put it on your fridge, bathroom mirror or pantry to help you remember how to interrupt greedy appetite, head or mouth hungers.**

**If you haven't already used the CPR audios then start today.**

| Remember your 10 Commitments |
|:---:|
| Rehearse Outfit |
| Audio Daily |
| Weigh Once |
| Stomach chooses |
| Smaller Portions |
| Chew Slowly |
| Push Plate |
| Thirst = Water |
| Wiggle Move |
| Write Progress |

# FOUR

## Control & Conquer Cravings

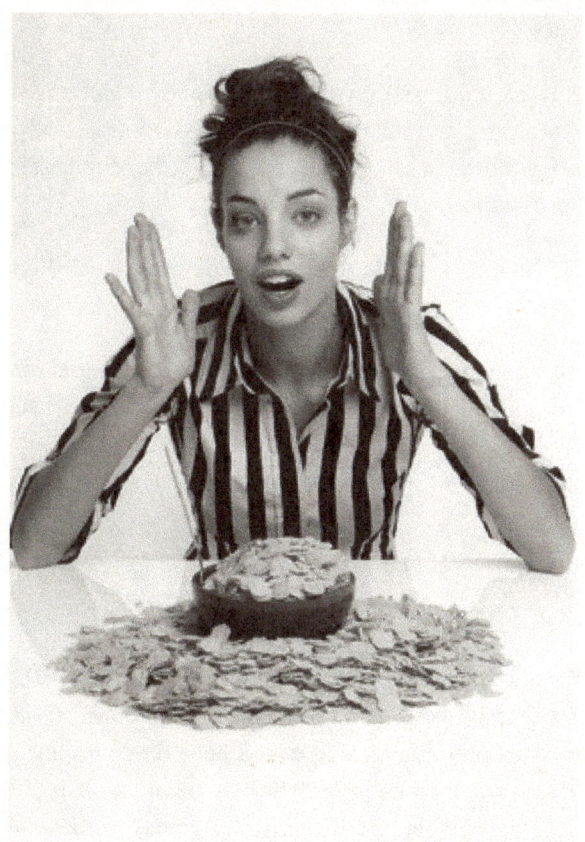

As you progress on your Unzip the Fat Suit journey, this Native American story can help you understand how important it is to change your thinking in order to achieve what you want.

**Which part wins? Is it the greedy wolf or the healthy dream?**

# THE TWO WOLVES
## *Traditional legend - original author unknown*

A Grandfather from the Cherokee Nation was talking with his grandson.

"A fight is going on inside me," he said to the boy. "It is a terrible fight and it is between two wolves. One wolf is evil and ugly: He is greedy, angry, filled with envy, self-pity, sorrow, regret, guilt, resentment; he is lacking in confidence, false pride, superiority and inferiority. At the same time he is selfishness and arrogance. He is this all at once."

"The other wolf is beautiful and good," he continued. "He is loving, friendly, joyful, peaceful, healthful and helpful. He is hope, serenity, humility, kindness, benevolence, justice, fairness, empathy, generosity, true, compassion, gratitude, and has a deep healthy vision."

"This same fight is going on inside you and inside every other human as well," said the Grandfather.

The grandson paused in deep reflection because of what his grandfather had just said. Then he finally asked; "Oyee! Grandfather, which wolf will win?"

The elder Cherokee replied, "The wolf that you feed."

This fight exists inside each of us. I spent years conflicted by which wolf to feed. When we feed the greedy wolf, then that part of us becomes stronger and more powerful. We feed that part by listening to and believing our unhelpful self talk, and we feel fear for how loud and powerful the greedy wolf is. We experience uncomfortable self doubt when we listen to the greedy wolf's lies. Those lies cause us to stay zipped in the fat suit and unhealthy, they cause us to move further from the goals we have for our health and our ideal weight and size.

When we feed the balanced healthy, stable wolf with healthy harmonious thoughts, a healthy way of eating, with new beliefs, with love and positive energy, with gentleness and compassion and then use the CPR audios, then the greedy hungry wolf, grows weaker and quieter, and the healthy wolf grows stronger and louder.

Which wolf do you allow to speak the loudest or go unchecked?

This metaphor is a wonderful example of the importance of being able to control the 'hungry greedy wolf' of cravings, toxic critical thinking, habitual eating and emotional connections to food. The more you continue to allow this thinking to go unchecked, the more challenging it becomes to unzip the fat suit.

This chapter is dedicated to showing you how to interrupt the greedy 'wolf' and feed the slim and healthy, kind, gentle, confident and passionate you. The loving and intelligent, wise and spirited you!

## Dealing with Boredom / Habitual Eating Appropriately

Throughout a typical day your brain and body have natural fluctuations in attention and energy levels. These fluctuations happen in regular cycles called **Ultradian Rhythms**. Everyone has these cycles.

These **energy and attention cycles** occur every 90 to 120 minutes. What this means is that your mind can naturally focus on a task and work with sustained energy for limited periods. Approximately after every 45-60 minutes we reach a peak, and for the next 45-60 minutes our attention and energy levels begin to gradually decrease.

During this natural decline in energy people often feel lethargic, sleepy and find it difficult to concentrate. This lethargy is interpreted by some as either boredom or the need to snack, pick or graze to indulge their sugar or caffeine cravings.

If at this time you chose instead to have a short energising break that stimulated your brain, then you would be able to refocus easily and begin a fresh 90-120 minute cycle of attention. You'd do this with increased productivity (and a reduced calorie intake).

It is important to disconnect the link between the brain's natural **downtime** and **the need to use food to fill the gap**. When you do this you can use **this natural downtime to *stimulate the mind and body in a positive and sustainable way instead.***

By taking a short break (10-15 minutes) after every 90-120 minute cycle then you become even more productive, more energised and enjoy your day more. Shift your posture, consciously stretch and take 6 deep belly breaths. By doing this you would ensure that you 'manage' your natural ***Ultradian Rhythms*** more effectively and not mistake them for 'boredom' or more unhelpfully, as a need for boredom eating.

## EVERYONE HAS THESE NATURAL CYCLES OF ENERGY AND FOCUS

### YOU ARE NOT BORED
*YOU ARE IN NEED OF HEALTHY STIMULATION*

### YOU ARE NOT HUNGRY
*YOU ARE IN NEED OF HEALTHY STIMULATION*

### YOU DO NOT NEED TO SNACK
*YOU ARE IN NEED OF HEALTHY STIMULATION*

- During these *downtimes* a slim and healthy person would naturally choose to have a glass of water, go outside for fresh air, go to the toilet, take deep breaths or do some stretching. They would use that time to walk, make that phone call, meditate, share a joke, talk and laugh and then get back to the job feeling more energised. (Notice all of the options mentioned were calorie free).
- The overeater/picker or habitual boredom eater on the other hand might use this *downtime* as an excuse for food. Over time cravings begin to develop to coincide with these cycles. The overeater or picker thinks it's because they need food, in reality, the brain simply needed a break and a little healthy stimulation.

*This explanation can help you understand your experience of cravings or urges with reference to **peaks and drops in focus throughout the day**. It helps you to see that you need to take responsibility during those peaks and troughs **to use Control audios or other short techniques from the book to break old habits**. It helps make you aware that when these natural downtimes occur, you need to create alternative slim and healthy ways to punctuate your day.*

*At first it may take your conscious effort and responsibility to use the Control audios to interrupt the neural connections associated with the habit. Eventually your brain starts to change for the better. You are free to choose healthier ways to deal with these natural peaks and troughs to renew your energy and focus.*

**Alternative ways to interrupt the drop in energy and focus and provide healthy stimulation**

- Drink water
- Make a herbal tea
- Walk away from the desk and stretch
- Use a Control audio or tapping technique to interrupt the pattern
- Take 6 deep belly breaths
- Mind Rehearse wearing your goal outfit
- Share a joke / connect with someone who is positive and refreshing
- Think about your most important reasons for slim and healthy (your 'why')
- Watch something that makes you laugh (I have about 5 or 6 YouTube clips on my phone and computer that make me laugh no matter how often I see them. When I need a break I watch one and have a glass of water. Laughter is one of the best ways to stimulate healthy energy and circulation to your organs and brain (and it burns kilojoules too!)
- Meditate by focusing on your breath for 10 minutes
- Use a Rewire audio (they only take about five minutes)
- Use 3 suggestions from the 'Power of Three' List

These drops in energy cycles **do not happen because** of a craving or need for food, they happen **because the brain naturally needs a break to feel stimulated and re-energised again**.

You have the ability and the solutions to interrupt the link between 'boredom' and food - it is simply up to you to use those solutions until a healthier pattern has been formed.

## *SUMMARY*

- The picker or overeater habitually responds to these drops in energy cycles by eating; the slim and healthy eater chooses to stimulate and energise their body with movement or healthy choices instead.
- When not aware that these natural **Ultradian Rhythms occur, boredom eaters** can be heard to say "I feel bored, I need something to eat" or "I need energy, I'll have something to eat". Or "Once I eat something I'll be able to get back to it."

- 'Boredom' can be solved by changing your **posture and energising the brain and body by doing something stimulating and different for a few minutes.**
- By recognising these 90-120 minute attention cycles and choosing to do something different you will re-energise your body, and your mind will naturally re-focus.

## Control and Conquer Cravings and other unhelpful issues

Feeling in control of eating patterns and cravings is easier when you use the Control audios and / or follow the Control demonstration videos on my YouTube channel *http://www.youtube.com/MaggieWilde*

**These simple audios and the craving control tapping exercises outlined in this chapter help you put a stop to:**

- Unhelpful Cravings (sugar, breads, salts, chocolates and more)
- Unhelpful Emotional States (emotional eating - 'granny's biscuit cuddle)
- Unhelpful Behaviours (picking, snacking, bingeing and more)
- Unhelpful Sensations (phantom head or mouth hungers)
- Unhelpful Thoughts (inner critic, judgment, obsessive food thoughts/ images)

**The Control audios draw upon a therapeutic technique called Meridian Tapping – let's look at what it is and how it works.**

When you have an urge for something sweet or savoury, the Control audios and exercises interrupt the electrical impulse in the brain that caused the craving.

Lets pretend for example that today you felt hurt by something someone said to you. This 'hurt' trigger causes a neural pathway to activate in the brain that had previously been triggered by hurt feelings. In the past, it was also only satisfied (switched off) when you ate something sweet or savoury.

For example if Granny's biscuit cuddle program is still operating, then that electrical circuitry is activated by the hurt feelings. Consciously you don't know why you reach for a chocolate biscuit, but the thought, craving and emotional desire for the biscuit is automatically stimulated. That neural pathway (that urge) only stops once you satisfy the craving. It then becomes dormant waiting to be triggered to 'help' you next time you feel hurt.

When you use the Control audios and tapping exercises you interrupt the link between the external trigger (the hurt feeling) and the electrical current that creates the craving. If the trigger no longer stimulates that neural pathway, the craving can no longer happen.

For example:

**Scenario Trigger:** Someone says something hurtful to you, or perhaps you are home alone and bored. You don't use the tapping Control techniques and the old craving occurs.

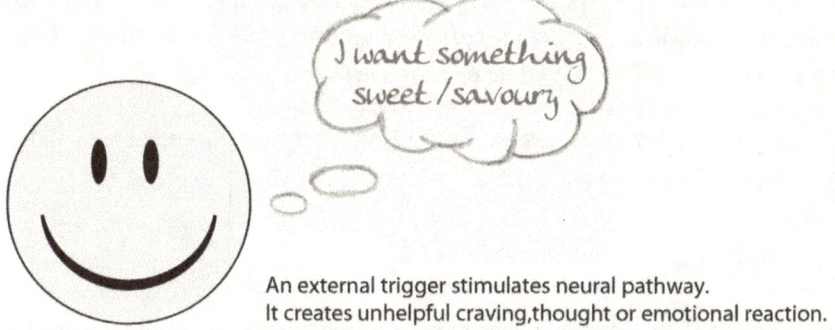

An external trigger stimulates neural pathway.
It creates unhelpful craving, thought or emotional reaction.

**Scenario Using Tapping and audios:** If the same 'trigger' occurs and you use the Control audios or tapping exercises, you interrupt the neural pathway that caused the craving or head hunger. You literally cannot hold the same thought or desire the same thing, in the same way. The energy or electrical charge is diminished, it is as though you turned off the switch and the neural pathway that stimulated the thought or craving, loses its strength.

When you use the tapping techniques the thought, feeling or craving changes.
You take control

**This means that:**

- When you use Control Audios in response to unhelpful food cravings *you can say instead: "I don't need that food"*
- When you use Control Audios in response to unhelpful feelings/emotions you can say instead: *"I don't feel the same way"*
- When you use Control Audios in response to unhelpful behaviour *you can say instead: "I don't need to do that"*

The Meridian Tapping technique used in the Control audios helps relax your brainwaves to a calm alpha state. Variations of this technique have been used therapeutically worldwide to help people overcome addictions, fears and phobias, post traumatic stress (PTSD) and other emotional issues.

I have provided a few versions of these techniques as both audios and video demonstrations for you to master.

## Control audios

There are quite a few different versions to download. Listen and follow word for word.

These techniques will help you control any unhelpful habit, emotional state or reaction as it happens. The techniques work instantly. In the meantime remember you are using the Program and Rewire audios daily to continue rewiring your mind for slim and healthy permanently.

- Control audios / videos and techniques achieve instant short to medium term control (for some people Control techniques, when used regularly, can create permanent change too)
- Program and Rewire audios achieve long term, permanent change

The demonstrations and audios ask you to tap or rub on meridian end points on the face and hands. By doing this you interrupt the electrical circuitry in the brain and diffuse any unhelpful reaction, thought or emotion associated with the unhelpful trigger and craving.

I also ask you to repeat certain statements while tapping on those points. (The Control Audios guide you through where to tap and what to say word for word). When you do this, you make a shift into a relaxed state, you stop the craving in its tracks.

In this state you experience a spontaneous relaxation of the conscious mind and a calming of the nervous system. The craving, emotion or thought that stimulated the desire for food simply dissolves because the electrical impulse has been 'switched off' from the neural pathway causing it.

## The hungry wolf no longer needs feeding

You no longer think, feel or wish to behave in the same way as before. Your brain no longer sends out the thoughts or Neuro-chemicals that caused the craving in the first place.

## The Benefits You'll Experience by using the Control Audios and Techniques

- You will feel more in control instantly
- You can adapt the technique for all purposes including unhelpful thoughts, behaviour, habitual eating, emotional eating, addictions, other unhelpful emotional states
- You can diffuse any trigger/craving/emotional state in moments
- You will instantly feel calmer and more positive
- You will stop repetitive/obsessive thoughts and create a 'quieter' mind
- You will reduce anxiety and stress
- You will stop unhelpful emotional reactions
- You will diffuse fear, anger and other unhelpful emotional states
- You will diffuse self doubt and develop self belief

**The tapping points: (Refer to the diagram and simply listen and follow the Control audio word for word)**

## Stage 1: Face and chest points

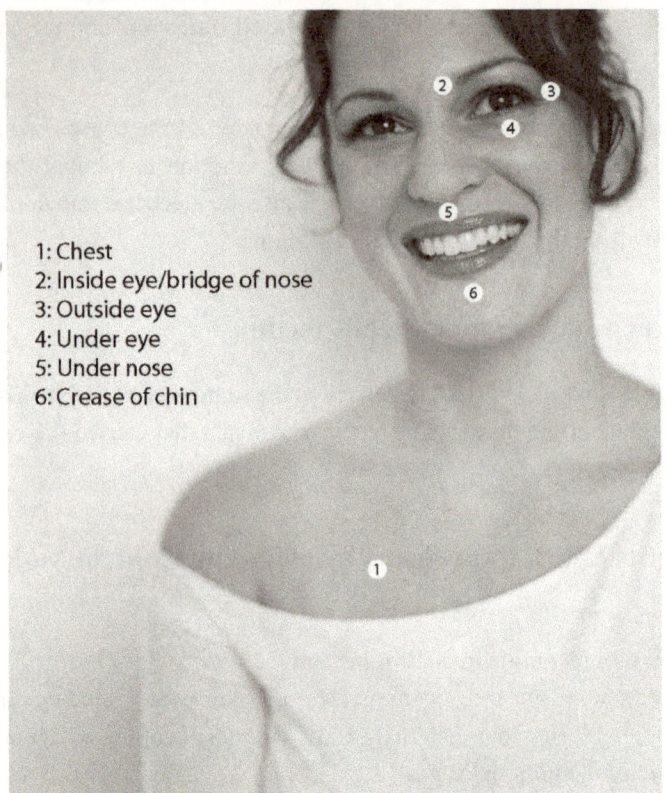

1: Chest
2: Inside eye/bridge of nose
3: Outside eye
4: Under eye
5: Under nose
6: Crease of chin

## Stage 2: Hand points

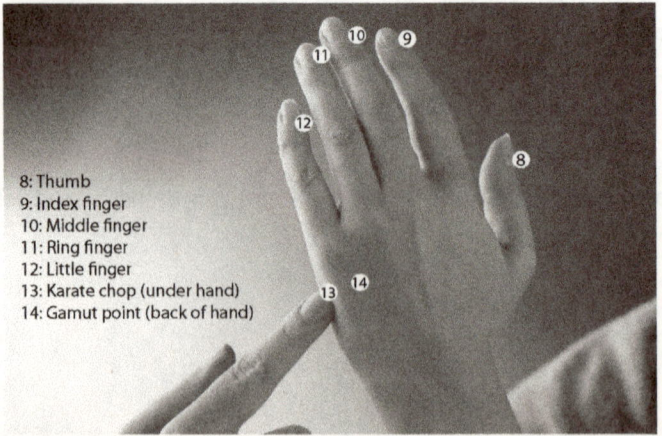

8: Thumb
9: Index finger
10: Middle finger
11: Ring finger
12: Little finger
13: Karate chop (under hand)
14: Gamut point (back of hand)

## Final Stage: Eye Movements (if required):

- Roll eyes up right
- Roll eyes up left
- Roll eyes down right
- Roll eyes down left
- Roll eyes in a circle one way
- Roll eyes in a circle the other way

When you listen to the audios or watch the video demonstrations, the specific sequence to tap on and what to say as you tap, are recorded word for word. All you need to do is – tap along and repeat after me.

## Short Cheat Sheet and an instant Craving Buster

Once you have learned how to do the tapping techniques by either listening to the Control audios or watching the demonstration videos, you can use shorter versions of these strategies without having to listen to the audios. To do this, I have designed a **Short Cheat Sheet** that can be done at home or at the office without having to follow the audios or videos. Once you know how you'll have an instant way to dissolve cravings wherever you are. I also have designed an instant **Craving Buster** for the moments when you just need help now! (Refer to charts 1 and 2. I have provided audio samples and video demonstrations of these for you to see how quick and simple they are: http://www.youtube.com/MaggieWilde

## Short Cheat Sheet – Chart 1

*(A brief demonstration video is available on the Youtube link above)*

Step 1: Assess the intensity of the unwanted feeling/craving on a scale of 0-10 (10 being the worst)

Step 2: Rub on the 'Sore spot' – (chest) and say x 3:

*"Even though I have this (craving/feeling.) I'm learning to love & approve of myself"*

(As you tap or rub on each point you will be saying the thing you wish to eliminate e.g. *craving, feeling)*

| Tapping Position | | *What to Say* |
|---|---|---|
| 1 | Tap inside eye *(bridge of the nose)* | *"this craving /feeling"* |
| 2 | Tap outside eye | *"this craving /feeling"* |
| 3 | Tap under eye | *"this craving /feeling"* |
| 4 | Tap under nose | *"this craving /feeling"* |
| 5 | Tap crease of chin | *"this craving /feeling"* |
| 6 | Tap chest | *"this craving /feeling"* |
| 7 | Tap thumb (by the nail) | *"this craving /feeling"* |
| 8 | Tap index finger | *"this craving /feeling"* |
| 9 | Tap middle finger | *"this craving /feeling"* |
| 10 | Tap ring finger | *"this craving /feeling"* |
| 11 | Tap little finger | *"this craving /feeling"* |
| 12 | Tap karate chop…as you say: | ***"I let this feeling /craving go. I let it go, I feel calm. Enough is enough, I feel good"*** |

- Take three deep breaths and as you breathe out say "I let it all go"
- Check the intensity now on a scale of 0-10
- If the rating is above a 1 it means there is still some of the unwanted feeling left…
- If so, tap on the Karate chop point and then continue by using the points and eye movements below

| 13 | Tap on Gamut point *(back of the hand between the last two knuckles)* | ***"I let this feeling / craving go… I let it go, I feel calm"*** |
|---|---|---|
| 14 | Keep your head still as you use your eyes to look up to the right | *"this craving /feeling"* |
| 15 | Keeping still, look up to the left | *"this craving /feeling"* |
| 16 | Look down to the right | *"this craving /feeling"* |
| 17 | Look down to the left | *"this craving /feeling"* |
| 18 | Roll the eyes in a full circle one way | *"this craving /feeling"* |
| 19 | Roll the eyes in a full circle the other way | *"this craving /feeling"* |

| 20 | Tap on the karate chop position again | *"I let this feeling /craving go... I let it go, I feel calm. The Past is the past, enough is enough, I move on, I move forward, I am stronger everyday"* |
|----|----|----|

- Take three deep breaths and as you breathe out say "I let it all go"
- Check the intensity now on a scale of 0-10
- If the craving is gone then enjoy your healthy day
- If there is any unwanted feeling left...
- Repeat the whole process above until you feel in control of the unhelpful craving/feeling

**Remember: use the demonstration audios and videos and practice till you feel in control of how to do this yourself with or without the audios.**

## Instant Craving Buster – Chart 2

*(A brief demonstration video is available on the Youtube link mentioned earlier)*

**Take a moment to assess the level of unhelpful craving or feeling on a scale of 0-10 (10 being the worst).**

**Tap on the chest point as you say:**

*"Even though I have this (craving/feeling.) It's time to let it go!"*

(As you tap on each point you will be saying the thing you wish to eliminate e.g. *craving, feeling*)

| | Tapping Position | What to Say |
|----|----|----|
| 1 | Tap under nose | *"this craving /feeling"* |
| 2 | Tap crease of chin | *"this craving /feeling"* |
| 3 | Tap thumb (by the nail) | *"this craving /feeling"* |
| 4 | Tap index finger | *"this craving /feeling"* |
| 5 | Tap middle finger | *"this craving /feeling"* |

| 6 | Tap ring finger | *"this craving /feeling"* |
|---|---|---|
| 7 | Tap little finger | *"this craving /feeling"* |
| 8 | Tap on the karate chop point…as you say: | "I let this feeling /craving go. I let it go,  I feel calm. Enough is enough, I feel good" (repeat x 3) |

Take three deep breaths and as you breathe out say "I let it all go"

- Check the intensity now on a scale of 0-10
- If the craving is gone then enjoy your healthy day
- If there is any unwanted feeling left…
- Repeat the craving buster again

**To control and interrupt habitual and emotional cravings you can also use some of the techniques I provided earlier in the book on the:**

## Power of Three List

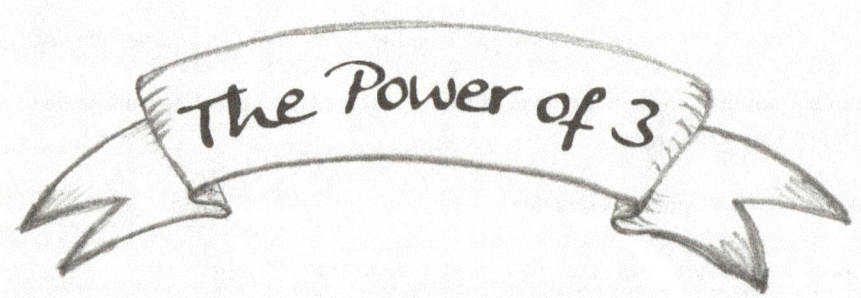

**An extended version of this list is provided below and will be the one you download if you wish to print it to use as a reminder at home. All of the techniques you have already learned, and a few others you will experience later in the book have been added. These will help you stay in control of what, when, why and how much you eat.**

## Craving Control Summary

Now that you understand the Control audios, I want to remind you of all the things you can do so far to interrupt cravings as you begin to rewire for slim and healthy.

If you suspect that greedy appetite, boredom hunger, head hunger, mouth hunger or some other emotional, habitual or stress 'hunger' is tricking you into thinking you are hungry, then simply commit to doing at least three of these steps before using food. This will help you feel more in control.

## The Power of Three Comprehensive List

**Do at least three of these steps**

1.  Use a Control audio, the Short Cheat Sheet or the Craving Buster
2.  Watch a demonstration video
3.  Have a glass of warm or room temperature water (with a squeeze of lemon or lime if you wish)
4.  Do 6-10 deep belly breaths
5.  Acknowledge that the feeling will pass. Experience it with amusement as you tap on the karate point and say *"I am in control, enough is enough"*
6.  Use the 'ask-answer-discuss' questions in chapter 3, then make a conscious decision whether to respond or reject it. To help with this use Control audios or the Craving Buster
7.  Ask yourself the Inner Coach questions in Chapter 5
8.  Use one of the Program audios (Eliminate Greedy Appetite or other)
9.  Use a Rewire Audio (Rewire for Slim & Healthy - Unzip the fat suit or other)
10. Use the Program audio 'Be Stress Free'
11. Use one or more of the techniques to reduce stress in Chapter 12
12. Mind Rehearse your 'goal outfit', imagine as if it fits already
13. Do something to move your body and stimulate endorphins for 10 minutes. For example go for a walk, dance, stretch, do a yoga pose as you repeat the phrase "enough is enough"
14. Think about your most important reasons for being slim and healthy as if it is real right now. Ponder your 'Why' and let yourself feel it, experience it with all of your senses as if it is already real
15. Write about the importance of your 'Why' in your progress journal (see Chapter 14)
16. Think about a time in your life where you showed determination and strength, really remember how it felt and how proud you were of yourself as if it is happening again today. (If you feel challenged to think of a time when you felt proud or strong, make one up or think of a time you felt proud watching a successful achievement of someone you care about)
17. Imagine being your ideal weight and size now. Feel, see, pretend as if it's real now, do it with all of your senses

18. Wiggle and move for 60 seconds: stand up and sit down, stretch, play your favourite tune and wiggle it, do star jumps, shake your body vigorously

19. Do the 'I'm Gorgeous: You're Gorgeous technique or any of the other techniques from Chapter 7

20. Repeat to yourself: "It's my choice. I can choose to feed the greedy wolf or the healthy me"

21. Ask the P.I.G. question *"Is this mouthful satisfying nutritional, habitual or emotional needs?'* (Refer to Chapter 6)

22. Remind yourself about how easy it is to break the habit of 'instant gratification'. Repeat in your mind: *"I choose to say no to ... (e.g. chocolate) now and if I want to, I can make a different choice tomorrow. Enough is enough, I'm in control"*

**Remember if you still have the unhelpful craving or emotion after genuinely committing to do at least three of the above it will be genuine appetite so...**

- Eat a very small amount of something nutritious such as nuts and seeds, a few grapes (only the amount that fits into the palm of your hand)
- To help the brain register that you have given the body nutrition eat slowly, chew consciously. Be aware of each mouthful as you bring it to your mouth, watch the food disappear from the palm, be aware of the textures and flavours in the mouth. (Refer to Chapter 8)

| **Remember your 10 Commitments** |
|---|
| Rehearse Outfit |
| Audio Daily |
| Weigh Once |
| Stomach chooses |
| Smaller Portions |
| Chew Slowly |
| Push Plate |
| Thirst = Water |
| Wiggle Move |
| Write Progress |

# FIVE

## Control & Conquer Unhelpful Thoughts, Emotions & Behaviour

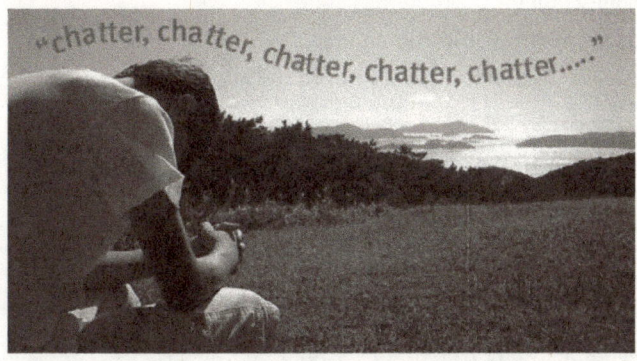

"chatter, chatter, chatter, chatter, chatter...."

In Chapter 2, I stated that to succeed at any goal you must have a plan. I outlined the 10 Commitments as the basis of your plan. In this chapter I delve a little deeper into how to put that plan into action.

In order to do this, we must assess and change any unhelpful beliefs, critical self-talk or emotional reactions that stop us from making healthy decisions about food and our body. When we do this, we can then have more space in our head for healthy thoughts about our body and ourselves, and more focus and motivation for healthy actions and habits too.

To succeed at unzipping the fat suit permanently, there may be times when you are faced with hurdles that cause you to doubt yourself or your commitment to your goal. Distractions, unhelpful or unsupportive people, events and circumstances do arise. The difference now will be that you can develop strategies to help you stay focused, no matter what distraction or hurdle you face. *To succeed you need contingency strategies* to overcome challenge and adversity along the way.

## Contingency Strategies to program and rewire permanently for slim and healthy

To permanently program and rewire for slim and healthy, it is important to address the following six steps:

1.  Use the CPR audios
2.  Follow your 10 Commitments

As strategies 1 and 2 have already been covered I will use this chapter to discuss points 3 to 6)

3.  Let go of Limiting /Unhelpful Beliefs
4.  Manage Unhelpful Emotional States
5.  Change Unhelpful Behaviours/Habits
6.  Eliminate Limiting or Unhelpful Self-Talk

Lets address limiting or unhelpful beliefs that held you zipped in the fat suit for too long.

## 3. Let go of Limiting /Unhelpful Beliefs

In life, we accumulate lots of helpful wisdom and experiences, however we also accumulate lots of unhelpful, out of date information too. You can learn something at one stage in your life that is a useful belief, however, later that belief may be out-dated, and it might even be unhelpful to you in achieving your current objectives.

**Example 1:**

You may have recognised as a child, that when you finished everything on your dinner plate, you were praised. Later, that awareness became a habit, and that habit eventually became a subconscious belief that says: *"I must always eat everything on my plate"*.

Much later as an adult, you may wish to change that habit so that you can act upon 'fullness' and push the plate away, rather than continuing till your plate is empty. People often find those habits challenging to change because the belief that causes the habit is still in place. That belief has become a subconscious 'lie' that you tell yourself because it is no longer based on fact. As a child, the fact was that you did get praised for finishing dinner, as an adult you no longer need that praise, but 'the lie' subconsciously urges you to continue the habit.

Internal conflict arises: *"I want to stop eating once I feel full, but I just keep eating till it's all gone"*.

**Example 2:**

If as a child you were told: *"it's only puppy fat, you'll wake up one day and it will be gone"*. You may now hold the unconscious belief (lie) that, *"I don't need to do anything, because one day I'll wake up and the fat will be gone"*. This can lead to patterns and habits of procrastination to move your body, or the lack of will to change your unhealthy habits. We are aware consciously we need to move our body or eat differently, but our subconscious as yet, does not believe this.

To unzip the fat suit permanently, it is important to regularly assess any unhelpful beliefs (lies) that your subconscious still holds onto. I recommend that you begin to notice unhelpful habits or thoughts and when you recognise them, ask yourself:

*"Am I holding onto any underlying beliefs (lies) that cause me to continue thinking or behaving in this way?"*

Once you notice these, then you can begin to program and rewire new, more helpful beliefs.

The first step is to recognise if there are any potential hidden 'fat suit' beliefs (lies) that might be holding you stuck in the fat suit. These subconscious beliefs or decisions we have previously made about ourselves, can be repeated so often that you no longer question them, and assume they are true.

In order to recognise any unhelpful beliefs you need to look out for *specific words* and phrases that should send alarm bells ringing. When I hear clients say these words or phrases I immediately stop and ask them: *'Who says?' Whose belief is that? Is this belief still relevant to you?'*

**Listen out for these alarm bells**

*I can't, I have to, I'm not, I couldn't, I'll never, I'm always, I don't, I doubt or I shouldn't.*

If you hear yourself say any of these take a breath and pause. These phrases will be the key you need to discover obsolete or false beliefs that keep you locked in the fat suit. These beliefs could be psychological and emotional barriers that keep you from your ideal weight, shape and size.

If you hear yourself say any of these alarm bell words or phrases' ask:

*'Whose belief is that?'*

*'Is this belief still relevant to me?'*

We often hold onto limiting beliefs that we 'learned' from parents, schoolteachers, friends or caregivers. These 'beliefs' might only have been opinions that you repeated endlessly to yourself for years. They might not have been true then, and certainly might no longer be true or serve your needs now.

An example of this could be our attitude about exercise or belief in our skills or intelligence. Some people hold beliefs or perceptions about their physical and intellectual capabilities based on something that happened at school or early in childhood (like the examples I mentioned earlier).

As an adult, these 'beliefs' will restrict how that person now responds to opportunities for exercise, health or intellectual capacity today.

It is important to regularly do a 'belief de-clutter', to shed the excess baggage of limiting beliefs.

The important thing to realise about beliefs is that people perceive them to be facts when in truth they are only perceptions, potentially based on someone else's opinion. These 'beliefs are accumulated from our current knowledge, past experiences and the attitudes or opinions of important authority figures in our life. They also include ideas or opinions expressed in what we read in the paper, or on social media, what appears on the web or what we hear on the news or from the latest gossip chain.

Until we do our own analysis to assess whether that belief is a helpful personal truth that we wish to keep, or a perception learned from someone else, we might consider that it requires more thought before we believe it or continue acting upon it.

Importantly, these past perceptions are stored in an area of your brain called the amygdala. For non-technical ease let's call this area in your brain the *'Perception Library'*. Take a minute to imagine it now, a little room in the front of your brain. It's filled with shelves like a library; each shelf stores the classification of all your life's perceptions. "This one is good", "Nope, that one is bad" and so on.

Every event, interaction, person or thing you have ever experienced is classified on those shelves as either something to feel safe about, or something to fear. Your brain's *'Perception Library'* classified each experience or interaction based on the memories that your brain has. Your *'Perception Library'* is always ready to communicate to another part of your brain that produces the Neuro-chemicals that cause emotional responses.

Let's call this other part of the brain, the *'Pharmacist'*. Its job is to release the right mix of chemicals to calm, motivate or stress you, based on your *'Perception Library's'* interpretation. Depending on which chemicals the *Pharmacist* releases you will have specific physical, emotional and/or physiological reactions.

You can read more about how to reprogram and rewire your brain's *Perception Library* and *Pharmacist* in relation to motivation to exercise in Chapter 9.

For now, it's simply important to understand, that these perceptions are stored in the library. The good news is, if the perceptions stored are unhelpful to you, then they can be de-cluttered and eventually changed. In this chapter, I will help you begin the process of de-cluttering the unhelpful perceptions and beliefs (subconscious lies) that hold you stuck in the fat suit. Used regularly, the CPR audios can then help to change them.

Make a list of the current limiting beliefs that may have kept you stuck in the fat suit.

These might include:

- I can't change, it's just the way I am
- I'm not good enough
- I'm not sporty
- I don't deserve to be healthy
- I'm not worthy
- I don't like exercise
- I can't lose weight easily
- I'll never be slim
- I'll always be fat
- I'm not slim enough
- I can't say no to chocolate/carbs etc
- I have to eat everything on my plate
- If others are having it I should have it too
- I'm lazy
- I don't like salad/vegetables/fruit

Tick any of the ones above that resonate with you and then add your own

- _____
- _____
- _____
- _____
- _____
- _____
- _____
- _____
- _____
- _____
- _____
- _____

Once you acknowledge these unhelpful beliefs it is important to ask:

- Whose belief is that?
- Is that belief still relevant to me?
- Is it helping me unzip the fat suit?
- Would I be willing to accept it as a past perception that I could change?
- If I was to change this perception, how would that change my life / body / actions?
- Is there anything stopping me from changing that perception/belief?
- Am I willing to use the Control audios to let it go?
- Am I willing to do that now? (if so, use the Control Feelings audio or video and exchange the word 'feeling' with the word, 'belief'.

*Remember:*

Step 1: Recognise unhelpful beliefs (be on alert for alarm bell words or phrases)

Step 2: Ask-answer-discuss the questions above (these questions are an example of the types of questions I use to deal with unhelpful beliefs

Step 3: Use the Control audios to interrupt the thought process and then re-assess whether you feel the same way. (As you tap on each point say *'this belief'*. When you get to the karate chop say *'I let this belief go, I don't need it anymore'*)

Step 4: Seek help if you recognise challenges that don't easily shift. Email me at info@thepotentialist.com

## 4. Manage / Release Unhelpful Emotional States

Unhelpful emotional states can limit us in a variety of ways too. Prolonged unhelpful emotional reactions such as anger, frustration and resentment, blame, rebellion, guilt, fear and jealousy can lead to lack of motivation, potential weight gain and slower weight reduction due to the release of excessive stress hormones. These unhelpful emotional reactions can also lead us to make bad decisions and take unhelpful actions, the results of which can end up being more disruptive to our life and body, if we need to undo or reverse those decisions or actions.

It takes an exhausting amount of energy to hold onto unhelpful emotions, so why not free that energy up and use it instead, for positive action to unzip the fat suit. When you remain in a negative state of mind, you produce lots of unhelpful stress hormones that exacerbate how you feel. Long-term, producing excess stress hormones will slow your weight reduction and, damage your physical health. By recognising how unhelpful this is to your body, you can begin to do something about it.

You can't control your outside world or how others behave or treat you; you can only control **how you react** to events, people and circumstances. So you might as well choose to react in a calm, resourceful, positive way, that supports you towards your ideal you.

When you are in an unhelpful state of mind, or reacting with an unhelpful emotional outburst or 'inburst' *(inburst is when we are emotionally responsive and we pretend to the outside world that we are not)*, then we produce those excess stress hormones I mentioned. (Refer to Chapter 12, which outlines the importance of stress management in relation to unzipping the fat suit).

Make a list of the unhelpful emotional states and reactions to people or events that affect your life in unhelpful ways. (Your outbursts and inbursts)

For example:

    a.   I get annoyed when people cut me off in traffic
    b.   I seethe when someone tries to tell me what to do
    c.   I feel pressured when people ask me questions or put me in the spotlight

    d.    (Person's name) always makes me feel nervous

    e.    I'm impatient when I wait in queues

    f.    I feel anxious if I don't have any sweets or chocolates in the house

    g.    I am scared I will never get this weight off

    h.    I'm depressed when I think about my body/weight

Tick or adapt any if they relate to you and add to your list:

1. _____
2. _____
3. _____
4. _____
5. _____
6. _____
7. _____
8. _____
9. _____
10. _____

When you become aware of unhelpful emotional reactions, outbursts or inbursts, it is important to ask:

- Whose reaction is this; did I learn it from someone else?
- Is reacting this way helping me unzip the fat suit?
- Am I willing to convert this unhelpful energy into more useful positive action? (E.g. convert anger into motivation to take action)
- Am I willing to use Control audios to interrupt this unhelpful emotional state?
- If I was to change this reaction how would that change my actions or my life?
- Is there anything stopping me from changing this reaction?
- How would my life/body/health be different if I let this reaction go?
- Am I willing to do that now?

Remember by changing your unhelpful reactions and emotional states, it doesn't make the behaviour, person or event right, it just means you no longer let them or it, hold you in the fat suit anymore. You control your life; the person, event or circumstance no longer controls you.

*Remember:*

Step 1: Be willing to recognise unhelpful emotional states (don't judge them, simply acknowledge them

Step 2: Interrupt them by doing the 'ask-answer-discuss' questions above

Step 3: Use the Control & Conquer Feelings audio or watch the demonstration video and shift your emotional state

Step 4: Use any other CPR audio of your choice to change your state

Step 5: Seek help if you recognise challenges that do not shift (email info@thepotentialist.com)

## 5. Change Unhelpful Behaviours

We all have them or know someone who does - unwanted, unhelpful habits or behaviours that limit our success.

These can include procrastination, self-sabotage, indecision, laziness, rashness, overeating and under eating, too much alcohol and not enough water. Then there are addictive behaviours that zap your time and energy rather than add to your passion for life. These can include: unhelpful attractions to things like chocolate, carbohydrates, chips, take-away food, caffeine, processed sugars, fizzy sugary drinks, alcohol, smoking, bingeing, television, or even other people's business. This list could go on. I'm sure you recognise at least one of these in yourself or someone you know.

For some people, these behaviours consume so much energy and time. If they are not doing them, they may be thinking about ways to do them, or beating themselves up about having done them.

To develop an attitude for slim and healthy permanently, it is important to recognise behaviours and habits that no longer help you. Your valuable time and energy could be better spent doing your 10 Commitments or an audio instead.

Sometimes changing unwanted behaviour is as simple as making the decision to stop. For some people, once they are aware of the unhelpful behaviour and they have prioritised their health and body and planned and set their goals, then stopping can be a simple choice.

For other people, stopping those behaviours and habits can be more challenging because internal conflict, or subconscious patterns may be at play. If this is the case, it will take commitment and persistence to use some of the following techniques and others throughout the book, to stop the behaviours. It is important to be honest with yourself, acknowledge that those behaviours exist, and start using your CPR audios daily.

Make a list of your unhelpful habits and behaviours that need to be interrupted in order to unzip the fat suit. (choose any from the ones I mentioned, if they are relevant, and add your own here)

1. _____
2. _____
3. _____
4. _____
5. _____
6. _____
7. _____
8. _____
9. _____
10. _____

Once you acknowledge an unhelpful behaviour or habit exists, it is important to 'ask-answer-discuss' using these questions:

- Is this behaviour or habit helping to unzip the fat suit?
- Would I be willing to use the Control audios to dissolve the unhelpful reaction to this habit, or the urge or craving that leads to the habit?
- If I were to change this behaviour to a more helpful one, what would I do?
- Would I be willing to use the Program and Rewire audios more often?
- If I was to change this behaviour how would that change my body/life/ actions?
- Am I willing to do that now?
- Is anything stopping me from changing this behaviour?
- If there is resistance to stopping it, am I willing to replay the Control Feelings audio, replace the word 'feeling's, with 'resistance' and tap on letting the 'resistance' go.
- Is my 'Why' do I want to unzip the fat suit more important than the behaviour? (If not, take a moment to re-assess your 'Why'. Find a 'Why' that you are more emotionally motivated by)

- Close your eyes and imagine the 'part of you' that does the behaviour and the 'part of you that wants to stop it, sitting together to talk about the issue. Take it in turn to listen to each part. Use the part of you that is your 'inner coach' (refer to point 6) to mediate a healthy agreement that both parties are happy with.

*Remember:*

Step 1: Be honest with yourself about unhelpful behaviours

Step 2: Interrupt the urge to do the behaviour or the behaviour itself by holding an internal discussion - use the questions above

Step 3: Use the CPR audios as recommended

Step 4: Use the Program and Rewire audios as recommended

Step 5: Regularly assess your 'Why'

Step 4: Seek help if you recognise challenges in letting unhelpful behaviour go (email info@thepotentialist.com)

## 6. Eliminate Negative or Unhelpful Self-Talk

### Turn Your Inner Critic into Your Inner Coach

The problem with 'self-talk' (whether positive or negative) is that it always feels true. Even though our thoughts might often be biased or based on unhelpful past experiences, perceptions and beliefs, we assume those thoughts are facts when they are actually perceptions.

His Holiness, the Dalai Lama says *"....train your mind in a daily practice that weakens negative attitudes and strengthens positive ones."*

It is important to become conscious of negative, unhelpful thoughts as soon as they start, and replace them with more positive ones. The first step to rewire these thoughts is:

**Become conscious of your unhelpful self talk. Once you become more aware that it exists, commit to swap it instantly with more positive language.**

## You can do this by: Turning your Inner Critic into Your Inner Coach

If you become aware of unhelpful self-talk about yourself or anyone else (judgements) then ask yourself this *key question* instantly:

*What would my inner coach say or do instead?*

As Dr Caroline Leaf says 'If left unchecked unhelpful thoughts can create illness and fester into deeper issues.' In her book *Who Switched Off My Brain* she uses the analogy "good thoughts are like beautiful, lush and healthy green trees, while negative thoughts are like ugly, mangled, snarling thorn trees."

In the same book, she refers to research that shows how having positive thoughts and using positive words can lead *to significant structural changes in the brain's cortex in only four days*.

**How amazing is that?**

*You can physically see the structural changes in the brain within four days after you start using positive language and thoughts.*

*Four days is all it could take to start programming and rewiring your brain for slim and healthy. Can you commit to at least four days to start shifting how you think about, feel and see your world?*

Using the 10 Commitments, the CPR audios and other exercises both in this chapter, and in the rest of this book, will have a noticeable positive effect very quickly. Within a very short time, you'll *feel emotionally better* anyway, so you're more likely to continue using the Commitments and the audios. Hey presto! You'll start unzipping the fat suit easily before you know it! Then, the motivation to reinforce these new helpful ways of thinking and feeling to your long-term memory is easier. Hooray! Permanent change!

**The following examples help you address your own self-talk. These ideas will help you be more aware of unhelpful, energy depleting self-talk and retrain your mind to create more helpful inner encouragement.**

If you recognise any of these 'negative' self talk examples, use the techniques outlined to transform them into positive language, this way your brain can begin to help you feel more positive too.

When you recognise unhelpful self-talk ask the key questions:

1.  What would my inner coach say or do instead?
2.  What positive language could my inner coach use instead?

I have provided a few examples of how you might change unhelpful self talk (inner critic), to helpful self talk (inner coach) language.

| Negative Self-Talk Used (Inner Critic) | Positive Language to Rewire (Inner Coach) |
| --- | --- |
| The problem is … | The Challenge or Opportunity is … |
| I can't … | I can learn how to … |
| It's impossible … | It's possible, I choose to discover how to … |
| I should … | I choose to … |
| I failed … | I learned from that experience … |
| It's difficult … | It's easy once I know how … |
| It's only / just me | It's me |
| I'm useless/ hopeless at this… | I'm discovering how to improve at this … |
| What if I fail… | How can I succeed … |
| This is too hard … | This is a challenge I can learn to overcome … |
| This is too hard … | I can ask for help … |
| I can't do anything right … | I choose to give it a go and learn … |
| I'm too fat / old / stuck in my ways … | I choose to change my health today … |
| This will take forever … | Every day I am one step closer to my goal … |
| I might or I'll try … | I choose … |
| Take a few moments to consider any unhelpful self-talk language you have used in the past. Convert the critic into the coach by asking 'what would my inner coach say instead?' Become more vigilant, mindful of your language and thoughts from today, and your brain and body will thank you for it. | |

| Unhelpful Self-Talk (inner critic) | Helpful Self-Talk (inner coach) |
|---|---|
|  |  |
|  |  |
|  |  |
|  |  |
|  |  |
|  |  |
|  |  |
|  |  |
|  |  |
|  |  |
|  |  |
|  |  |

**Exercise: Add to that list as you become aware of any other unhelpful self-talk. Always find the positive language to replace it.**

*Remember:*

Step 1: Be on the alert for unhelpful Self-Talk (the inner critic)

Step 2: Interrupt it and change it. Replace it with positive language

Step 3: Ask 'What would my inner coach say or do instead?'

Step 4: Ask: Does this language feel 'heavy' or 'light' in my mind and body?

- If you are left with a 'heavy' sensation in your body or mind when you repeat the 'self-talk', the words will keep you in the fat suit.
- If the language feels light when you repeat it, then your mind and body will be processing it positively. You will be moving toward your goal.

Step 5: Use Rewire audios daily and fill your mind with positive language

Step 6: Seek help if you recognise challenges in letting persistent unhelpful self-talk go (email info@thepotentialist.com)

**Extra key - surround yourself with positivity too**

> Just as it is important to de-clutter your beliefs, emotional states, unhelpful behaviours and your negative self-talk, it is vital to surround yourself with positive people too. We have all come across them, friends, colleagues, authority figures and even relatives that zap your energy and always tell you why the things you plan *will not work*. It is important to be aware of:

- People who are not supportive of your desire to unzip the fat suit permanently
- People who persistently tell you "you can't" or " you shouldn't"
- People who distract, or try to entice you away from your goal
- Negative people who complain all the time, but resist change themselves
- People who zap your energy, but don't follow through or take responsibility
- People who secretly don't want you to succeed, and perhaps don't believe you can

**Once you acknowledge these people exist, it is important to ask yourself:**

- Is this person helping me move toward my goal?
- What would my inner coach inspire me to do or say to them?
- Am I willing to either not allow them to influence me, or let them go?
- If I ignore their influence or let them go, how would that change my life?
- What, if anything, is stopping me from ignoring their influence or letting them go?
- What would be different about my body and me, if I did not allow that person to influence me?

**Focus tip: Make a commitment to surround yourself with positive, helpful people. Be aware of interactions with people that leave you feeling depleted, exhausted or no longer motivated towards your goal. Extract yourself as soon as you can and do a Program or Rewire audio to change your thinking fast!**

If you require further help to address unhelpful self-talk, limiting beliefs, unhelpful emotional states and behaviours you can contact me on info@thepotentialist.com

---

*"Happiness depends more on the inward disposition of mind than on outward circumstances." Benjamin Franklin*

---

## A little story of my own

I want to share with you a story of my own because it highlights the important shift that happens when you change your thinking.

Years ago, I was living in London and I existed as half of a hapless and hopeless marriage that eventually ended with relief, for both parties. I had lost myself in that marriage, I was trying to be what I thought others wanted, and I was failing drastically, because I had stopped knowing who I was.

My aim had become: Be what I thought others wanted, in order to make them happy.

My ex-husband and his family were a close, strong unit. Each family member, including him, had a dominant personality. Early in our 'family relationship', I learned that my place within it was to listen. My opinions were not often heard, so I stopped offering them.

After a few years, I lost myself completely in a world where I became their 'perfect wife and daughter-in-law'. I smiled dutifully through it all, but deep within I had become bitter, angry and resentful.

I lost my confidence; I became resentful and blamed my ex-husband for how my life was. At that time, my thoughts were like toxic waste, just thinking about his lack of commitment to the relationship and everything I had 'given up' for him, made me seethe with dislike for him, and hatred for myself for staying. This was not a recipe for a healthy relationship at all.

Often the thoughts I had about him and myself, at that time, made me feel physically sick. My toxic thinking had depleted my confidence so much that I continued to stay in the relationship. This of course, didn't help either of us, as we were both desperately unhappy.

Thankfully, the marriage did eventually end, and despite the secret sense of freedom I felt when this happened, I was too scared to face the separation for *two reasons*.

The first reason was to do with an *old belief* that had also kept me tied to the relationship, and the second reason was to do with the toxicity of the previous unhelpful self-talk.

This self-talk had created in my mind, a black hole about the future. I couldn't contemplate the thought of staying in the relationship, but the fear of being alone was far more overwhelming.

The *first reason* was that, at that time, I had a belief that 'Being divorced was wrong'. I had grown up in a Catholic environment and had been indoctrinated with the belief that it was a sin to divorce. No matter how painful the marriage was to both of us, I had held onto this subconscious belief. As I contemplated the separation I could still hear my mother's words echoing in my mind *'You made your bed, you have to lie in it, it's your responsibility no matter how bad it is'*. As I realised this, I asked myself these questions: 'Is the church's and my mother's belief helping either him or me right now? Is this belief still relevant to me, and if not, what would happen if I let this belief go?'

The *second reason:* I was still too scared to face the separation because of my toxic self-talk. It filled my entire headspace. Even after we separated, I was living in London waiting for the sale of the property to be finalised and I was terrified of what the future held. I could not think positively about my future because there was no room in my head. I was aware of how bad the relationship and my life had been behind me, but I could not contemplate the prospect of a future. I was depressed, anxious and fearful, I didn't want to, nor could I go back to how it was, but I had no confidence to go forward.

I would cry and cry until I thought I couldn't cry anymore, and then I would cry some more. At night, I would wake in the empty apartment in a state of tangible fear, I would literally wake trembling. My mind would race and spin out of control. *"What if...?"*, *"where will I go?"*, *"how can I survive?"* and *"I was the marriage, I'm no-one without it"*.

This last thought, was the deal breaker for me. I realised one night as I sat bolt upright in bed, I was happier before the relationship started, I was miserable in it. D'oh! I had forgotten. I had stopped accessing all the goodness that was in me, all of the confidence, the strength, the happiness, the energy I had. I had learned new unhealthy ways of thinking in a short few years, which had over-ridden the good stuff. My mind had become so full of the toxic self-talk, that there had been no room to remember who I had been and how I had felt, before the relationship.

So I wrote myself a list that very night. This list was all I was capable of thinking that night. (I have since adapted this list, and I will show you how I amended it in a moment)

I am confident – I had forgotten and I remember that now

I am strong – I had forgotten and I remember that now

I am beautiful – I had forgotten and I remember that now

I am loving – I had forgotten and I remember that now

I am loved – I had forgotten and I remember that now

I am intelligent – I had forgotten and I remember that now

I am kind – I had forgotten and I remember that now

I enjoy feeling free – I had forgotten and I remember that now

I enjoy learning – I had forgotten and I remember that now

I am learning from this – I remember that now

I read and re-read that list every day so many times. I made lots of copies. I had one under my pillow in case I woke frightened in the night. I had a copy in my handbag. I had it on my bathroom mirror, on my fridge. I put one everywhere I could in order to re-awaken the joy I used to feel. Often at first, I had to invent or pretend the joy until I began to experience it for real. It was as though the toxic thinking and words that I had learned, had consumed me and changed who I thought I was.

That list, was the thing that kept me safe until I found my confidence and my spark again. Within a couple of weeks, the fear of change was simply a speck on the horizon, and I realised I was excited about my future. I had so many plans, and I am proud to say, those plans are evolving, even to this day.

**As my confidence grew again, I realised there was a flaw in the original list, so I amended it like this:**

## My I Am List

I am confident

I am strong

I am beautiful

I am loving

I am loved

I am intelligent

I am kind

I am creative

I am prosperous

I am joyful

I enjoy freedom

I enjoy connection

I enjoy learning

Whatever this is, I am learning from it

I still refer to this list regularly … I call it my 'I AM' List

**Exercise:**

Take a few moments to create your 'I AM' list, keep adding to it and adapting it as you remember who you are underneath the fat suit. Start to remember or create who you are underneath the unhelpful beliefs, thoughts, feelings and emotions. You were born with the potential of being a healthy, joyous, loving, gorgeous, uniquely gifted, slim and healthy person. So if the fat suit hides you from you, if the unhelpful self-talk (inner critic) has kept you from unzipping it, then it's time to discover this amazing you!

Take the time to consult your inner coach about writing your "I AM" list now!

| I am ... |
|---|
| I am... |
| I am... |
| I am... |
| I am... |
| I am... |
| I am... |
| I am... |
| I am... |
| I am... |
| I am... |
| I am... |
| I am... |

**In summary: it's time to discover the real you. To control and change anything unhelpful to you, anything that has kept you from fulfilling your slim and healthy potential.**

You are not your thoughts, you are not your beliefs, and you are not your emotions or behaviours. You are not even the body that you walk around in. If you were any of these things, then *who is the 'you'* that *observes or judges* all of those things?

You were born as a divine, perfect healthy spirited baby; no matter who you think you are you now, you were born this way. You learned how to be and do all of the behaviours, thoughts and emotions you now experience. You learned the beliefs that you now hold, and you learned your reactions to food, people, events and circumstances that you now have. You even learned how to be inside a fat suit. Is that still working for you?

If you learned all this, you can now learn how to unzip the fat suit permanently too.

You are simply a product of your past experiences and your perceptions of those experiences. By using the steps outlined, you can begin to take full responsibility for discovering the real, healthy, slim, beautiful, handsome, joyous and divinely spirited soul that is you!

**All things are changeable when you know how so:**

1. Use the CPR audios (we know why and how they work - use them!
2. Consult your Inner Coach everyday
3. Do a belief de-clutter regularly – change unhelpful beliefs with the tools in this chapter and the Program and Rewire audios
4. Manage unhelpful emotional states with the tools in this chapter and the CPR audios
5. Change unhelpful behaviour with the tools in this chapter and the Control audios first. Then follow through with the Program and Rewire audios to change behaviours permanently
6. Eliminate unhelpful self-talk (inner critic crap) by consulting your inner coach regularly throughout the day. Use the tools in this chapter and the Program and Rewire audios to create more positive thinking patterns permanently
7. Read and re-read your 'I AM' list every day. Feel it and see it with all of your senses.

| Remember your 10 Commitments |
|:---:|
| Rehearse Outfit |
| Audio Daily |
| Weigh Once |
| Stomach chooses |
| Smaller Portions |
| Chew Slowly |
| Push Plate |
| Thirst = Water |
| Wiggle Move |
| Write Progress |

# SIX

---

## Stop Eating Your Emotions – How to Disconnect Emotions and Food

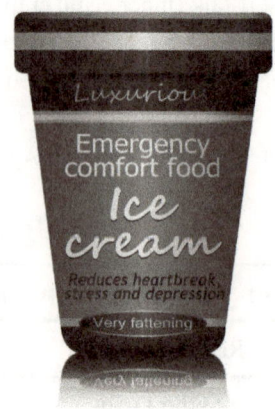

- Do you ever crave something sweet after dinner, even when you're already full?
- Have you ever reached for salty chips, a bottle of wine, a slab of cake, or some other 'treat' after a stressful argument or a bad day at work?
- Do you ever kid yourself by thinking: *just one more'* *'or* *'once it's gone I won't be tempted'* as you scoff biscuits or plough into a block of chocolate?
- Has half a cheesecake or a litre of ice cream disappeared, because you needed an emotional boost or a lift?
- Have you ever finished that bottle of wine and cheese platter, because you felt you deserved a break, or needed to numb the pain after a stressful week at work?
- Have you found yourself opening the fridge or pantry, looking for a treat when you're bored or lonely, or because you don't feel satisfied?

If you haven't, I'm sure you may know of a friend who has, perhaps they helped you down the wine, or scoop out the ice cream, while commiserating with you.

If that is the case, neither of you would be alone, because worldwide the relationship between food and emotions, eating, depression, anxiety and unhelpful stress or agitation, is very strong indeed. Understanding how emotions and stress trigger which comfort food you reach for, can help you make better choices and take deliberate control of how much you eat, and what and why you eat.

Importantly, as I mentioned in Chapter 3, understanding which emotional triggers and which stressful events cause you to reach for which specific snack foods, will be enormously helpful in breaking the habits and rewiring for slim and healthy.

Remember, your mind learns through repetition and heightened emotional states, so when you repeatedly do one action, while you are feeling a heightened, strong emotion; your brain connects the two things. It creates a link between which foods to crave, in order to satisfy which emotional state you're in. Funny about that, your mind can work for you, and against you, so let's learn how to control which way it wires from now on.

There is only one reason to create a love affair with food. That reason is because it is the source of your energy and health. It is the source of the vitality that allows you to bounce out of bed and live a long and active life, with those that you care about.

I've talked a little so far about potential unhelpful links between emotions and food. I want to address now, the importance of how to help your brain relearn that we eat only to fulfil the need for nutrition, that eating is no longer about 'eating or suppressing our emotions'.

In this chapter, I will address specific strategies to deal with, and break any unhelpful links between emotions, food and eating.

You were born needing to eat food with nutrients to keep your body healthy, to grow and be active; you were not born to eat emotions. When you repeatedly chew on emotions, swallowing them and stuffing them down, they eventually cause your body and mind, to become sick and toxic.

When you are stressed, depressed, angry, sad, resentful, rebellious, frustrated, fearful or anxious and you eat to make yourself 'feel' better, then you are literally eating your emotions. If you eat when you are in need of reward or punishment, or for any other reason on the emotional scale, then you are clogging your mind and fattening your body.

Perhaps that's why some people tend to overeat or binge when they eat their emotions, because no amount of food, no matter what it is, feels satisfying.

Guess Why? Emotions are invisible; when you eat them your brain can't 'see' what you're eating.

When you eat for emotional reasons, emotion overrides logic. You inhale the emotion (food), chew on it, suck it down, and hold it all together until you feel good again. It's as though you are holding your breath (ignoring logical inner coach thinking) the whole time.

**Guess what happens then?** When you finally stop gorging and chewing on those emotions, you feel worse. Oh yes, then the guilt and remorse flows. The *'I'm use-less, hopeless, there I go again'* thoughts and emotions take hold, proving that; yes indeed, you were right all along, you are a lost cause.

The cycle then continues: feel bad, eat more, and feel bad again…

When you eat due to stress or boredom, you also cause your body *and* mind distress in other ways. With boredom eating, you create more lethargy; slowing the brain's ability to focus and make logical decisions. You literally find it harder to think clearly and say "stop". With stress eating, you interrupt the digestive system and metabolic rate. You literally slow the weight reduction process down.

All of these emotional eating patterns immediately put your body into what is called the *fight, flight or freeze* response. One of the physical effects of the fight, flight or freeze (FFF) response, is that the energy your body would normally use for digestion, is diverted elsewhere in the body. This is useful if we need energy to run away from a tiger or hide from a threat, but it is not helpful for healthy digestion or to unzip the fat suit easily.

It is important to understand that it's time to 'love' food for the right reason. It's time to stop using food as a way to compensate for, or provide the comfort, acceptance, recognition or love that all humans need and deserve. To do this, we simply need to ask our inner coach the:

## P.I. Gauge – The P.I.G.

The P.I.G question is the gauge that will help you determine what type of hunger you are experiencing, and how to respond appropriately to it. So ask your inner coach the following P.I.G. question:

*"Is this mouthful satisfying nutritional, habitual or my emotional needs?"*

If you were being honest, more often than not, the answer would be habitual or emotional needs. Just by silently asking this question before the next mouthful of food, you could potentially eliminate lots of excess kilojoules every day.

Think about your breakfast, lunch and dinner. How often do you eat more than you need because it is on your plate? What about the snacks, morning or after-noon teas or after dinner sweets? If you were to ask the P.I.G. question halfway through each meal or snack: *"Is this mouthful satisfying nutritional, habitual or my emotional needs?"* then you could, more often, push the plate away, without needing to finish everything on it!

What are the emotional or habitual needs you are attempting to satisfy when you reach for excess food, comfort or stress food?

- Perhaps you're seeking time out to think and be you?
- Are you in need of connection, to no longer feel alone?
- Is it to feel safe or protected?
- Was it a need for love, or to feel comforted?
- Perhaps it was to feel accepted, heard, acknowledged or something else?
- Could it be a need to fill the gap of 'boredom'?

**What are you really looking for in that chocolate bar, or oversized bowl of pasta?**

Once you pause to ask the ***P.I. Gauge***, you discover more often than not, that it wasn't a family block of chocolate that your body or mouth wanted, it wasn't

129

really a kilogram of starch or a packet of stodge. What you really wanted was a hug, or you wanted to be heard, or to feel accepted or comforted in a moment of vulnerability or while in a heightened emotional state. You wanted to feel rested or peaceful, or you simply wanted to feel better than you did before.

You were seeking to lift the heaviness of unhelpful emotion, doubt or fear that you felt before you ate whatever it was that you ate. Instead, you felt worse because after the packet was empty, or the chocolate bar gone, you experienced heaviness in your stomach, you often felt guilt, remorse, regret and for some people, rejection of yourself or even, self-loathing.

> *The inner critic then bombards your mind with toxic chatter.*

> *"I can't believe I did that" or "I'm an idiot, here I go again".*

- It wasn't really four pieces of toast dripping with peanut paste that your lonely heart wanted, it was kindness, or a friend to talk to
- It wasn't really the giant pizza your eyes or head wanted; it was the connection with your friends, or the feeling of acceptance
- It wasn't really the bucket of KFC or the bar of chocolate that your hurt feelings needed. It was a cuddle, or a genuine listening ear

When you pause to treat yourself and your body with the respect, acceptance and the kindness that, deep down, you were seeking, you feel peaceful. When you recognise and offer yourself what you really needed and wanted; an *inner cuddle, time out* or a *genuine connection with a friend,* you feel full! When you provide the emotional support and appropriately fill your 'emotional hunger', then and only then, will you feel satisfied!!

When your brain finally rewires to understand that the purpose of food is to provide nutrition, the nutrients you need to be healthy, then the decisions about what, where, why and how much you eat, are effortless. Those decisions become congruent with your subconscious and your conscious desire to be healthy. No more inner conflict.

Once again, this is why the CPR Audios are so important in the journey you are undertaking. The audios help to Program and Rewire your mind so that you can choose healthier options, and smaller portions, easily from today and into the future.

If overeating, eating your emotions, stress, or habitual and binge eating has been an issue for you or someone you know, it is important to rewire your brain to love the fact, that food provides the nutrition for your body to live.

- **Emotional needs** *(emotional hunger)* **require** *compassionate, emotional responses* **to satisfy them**
- **Genuine hunger requires** *nutrition* **to satisfy it**

It is important to recognise those two distinct differences. To do this, we must disconnect the link between emotional needs and food, and make the connection between genuine hunger and nutrition.

If you have already started to use the CPR audios, and especially the Program and Rewire audios, you will already be helping to create a healthier outlook. Remember your neural pathways (brain patterns) start to rewire within days, making it easier to keep going once you make a start. The more often you use the audios, the better you begin to feel, and the better you begin to feel, the more likely you are to use the audios. You literally begin to handle daily emotional challenges, more easily.

To create a healthy relationship with food and your body, you must program and rewire your mind to choose healthier nutritious options, and to love every morsel you eat, *because it sustains your body.* Food *provides the energy* your body needs to reach it's potential. That does not mean that you will never eat a sweet or never indulge in your favourite treats again, what it means is that your mind will be rewired to know that *your primary reason* to eat, is to provide nutrition for your body to be energised and healthy. Having the 'occasional' treat is of far less importance.

*This simply means, you'll naturally want less of the treats, and reach for them less often.*

The main points so far:

- Respond to all types of hunger by asking the P.I.G. Question: *"Is this mouthful satisfying nutritional, habitual or my emotional needs?"*
- When the response is nutrition: make mindful choices about which foods you choose in order to provide the nutrition your body is asking for. Consult your stomach about which nutritious option to choose
- When the response is habitual or emotional needs, commit to using one of the Control audios, or remind yourself of the 'ask-answer-discuss' questions in Chapters 3 and 4.

- Disconnect emotional needs from food and eating by listening to the audios, completing the exercises and strategies throughout the book, interrupting the patterns with the 'Power of Three List'
- Remember:
  - Emootional needs require an emotional response (kindness, listening ear, hugs), that is the only way they will be satisfied
  - Nutritional needs require a nutritional response
- You can provide the kindness that emotional needs require by pausing, and listening to you, giving yourself an inner hug, or by picking up the phone to chat to a friend, instead of opening the pantry
- Use the Control audios to interrupt the pattern or connection between emotions and food, the Program audios to lay the foundation for the healthier neural pathways, and the Rewire audios to help make the change permanent
- Remember, it doesn't mean you can never have a treat again, it simply means you will rarely want them because your primary programming will be to provide nutrition for your body to live
- Take responsibility to provide the emotional support you need, you deserve to really satisfy this need once and for all
- Remember also, when you slow down and chew more, when you check in with your stomach between mouthfuls, and when you tunc in to the tastes and textures of each mouthful, you actually enjoy your food more anyway. When you enjoy your food more, you experience more satisfaction after far less food than before, meaning you consume less kilojoules anyway

## Quantity versus Quality

Whether you choose nutritious or unhealthy food, it is vital to always consider the importance of quantity too. Even healthy nutritious options can cause the brain to become overwhelmed, if you binge on them or over indulge.

It is important to tune into your stomach for that comfortable feeling between mouthfuls. Ask: what is the purpose of the next mouthful? Remember the client I mentioned earlier in the book who became stuck on a weight plateau? She was eating nutritious, healthy meals, but the portion size was *'supersize me'*. As soon as she reduced her portion size, the weight began to shift. If you choose the occasional treat consciously, for a particular reason, then it's simply about rewiring: *Less of it and less often – the CPR audios will help you do this.*

The connection between mood and food

As I've discussed previously, the reasons we reach for certain foods when we experience certain moods, is a combination of personal taste and learned chemical response in the brain and body. Certain foods literally impact the physiology of our body, and affect the stability of our emotional states. Some foods make us feel more alert, and others calm us down.

If you have habitually used certain foods to feel a certain way, your body and brain will send craving signals each time you feel that way. A habit can become an even stronger habit.

Brian Wansink, Ph.D. of Cornell University, suggests that if you want to feel relaxed and unwind, then having a carbohydrate rich snack will help the body feel as though it has relaxed. Used appropriately, this can be useful knowledge, however when used inappropriately, then you can develop unhelpful habits and reinforce the fat suit. Oh no!

Dr Wansink informs us that certain foods increase neurotransmitter production. Neuro-transmitters are the little chemical communicators that connect and communicate from one cell to the next in your brain and body. Some of these neurotransmitters literally excite or activate cells, and some will calm them down.

This chart from http://www.stonyfield.com provides examples of the effects that some foods have on neuro-transmitters and therefore, how those neuro-transmitters will make us feel.

| Nutrient | Food sources | Neuro-transmitters | Likely effect |
|----------|--------------|--------------------|---------------|
| Protein | Meat, dairy, eggs, cheese, fish, beans | Dopamine, Norepinephrine | Increased alertness, concentration |
| Carbohydrate | Grains, fruits, sugars | Serotonin | Increased calmness, relaxation |
| Excess calories | TOO MUCH of ALL foods, healthy or unhealthy, especially fat | Reduced blood flow to the brain | Decreased alertness, concentration |

## Food Coma

Overeating or ingesting too much food, no matter what it is, healthy or not, leads to a state of *food coma*. Food coma is a decrease in alertness causing us to feel as if we are sedated. Have you ever felt that '*I don't want to get off the couch lethargy*' after a big Sunday lunch? Has your stretched and aching belly made you want to lie down after eating too much? Remember, being slim and healthy is also importantly, about quantity of food, not simply quality of choice!

Can using the right foods to trigger the right moods (for example carbohydrates in small quantities to relax) be helpful?

Yes in theory. Unfortunately we often 'binge' on these foods as the mood takes control. The whole chocolate bar or four slices of toast is consumed before we force ourselves to stop. Rather than feeling in control of the mood, observing it, then doing something pro-active to change it, the mood controls you.

**Remember: never make a decision while in a bad mood; it will be a bad decision. This saying is especially true for decisions about food.**

If you are sad, depressed, grieving or lonely and craving your 'usual food fix', use Control Audios or the meridian tapping exercises from Chapter 4 to interrupt the pattern. Use at least 3 of 'The Power of Three' exercises or 'ask, answer, discuss' using the questions from previous chapters. Call upon your *inner coach* to help you discuss the trigger, pattern or reaction and choose a healthier alternative. Ask your *inner coach* the P.I.G question too. (Use the example 'ask, answer, discuss' questions in Chapters 3 and 5).

If the desire for food persists after you complete some of these tasks, it will be a genuine need for nutrition. In this case, eat a small handful of serotonin stimulating carbs such as fruit. It will help to genuinely lift your mood, while you continue using the tapping, CPR audios or other exercises to manage and rewire your reaction permanently.

*That is you being in control of the mood, rather than the mood, controlling you.*

Remember that overeating: eating beyond what your body actually needs, or eating when you are not genuinely hungry at all, eating too much of *anything (including healthy food),* causes a reduced blood flow to the brain and a decrease in energy and alertness. You'll enter a *food coma.*

I'm sure most of us at one time, have experienced that 'bloated' uncomfortable "I can't move" or "I wish I hadn't eaten all that" feeling that I've mentioned before.

**The keys to:**

Disconnecting the link between emotions and food

Disconnecting the link between unhelpful habits and food

Disconnecting the link between anything unhelpful and food

1. Use the Control, Program and Rewire audios regularly
2. Consult the 10 Commitments – complete the ones that need to be completed for the day
3. Use the Control audios and/or the short cheat sheet or the craving buster tapping techniques
4. Ask your inner coach the P.I.G. question before each bite: ***Is this mouthful satisfying nutritional, habitual or my emotional needs?***
5. Become mindful, observant of the triggers that stimulate different emotions that lead to the desire for specific mood foods
6. Do at least three of the 'Power of Three' techniques
7. Become mindful of the types of food you choose that will create the right chemical response in your brain and body (refer to the *stonyfield* chart)
8. Eat less of those old treats and choose them less often
9. Chew all food slowly and mindfully
10. Pause between mouthfuls, consult your stomach and listen out for the full feeling, repeat the phrase silently in you mind *'enough is enough'* after each mouthful until you feel ready to push the plate away
11. Seek professional help if you suspect an addiction is challenging your ability to change (email: info@thepotentialist.com)
12. Learn how to deal with adverse situations in different ways from today. Learn new reactions to triggers or old patterns. *(Increase your adversity quotient)*

**How will you deal with adversity / emotional upsets in the future?**

## Your Adversity Quotient

First there was IQ (Intelligence quotient), then there was EQ (Emotional quotient), now there is AQ your (Adversity quotient).

AQ is a rating that tells you how well you deal with adversity or challenge. Often people who have been persistent emotional or stress eaters, will have some work to do to rewire and increase their AQ levels. This is important so that your reactions to everyday challenge and adversity can be more helpful and healthful to you. If you learned to turn to food to cope when something went wrong in the past, then the CPR audios will definitely help boost your AQ. They'll help you deal with challenge more appropriately from today.

## What is AQ?

AQ was originally devised by Paul G Stoltz in 1997. In his book *'Adversity Quotient: Turning obstacles into opportunities'*, Paul defines AQ as *"The capacity of the person to deal with the adversities of life. As such it is the science of human resilience."*

Someone with a high AQ handles adversity or challenge by finding ways to appropriately and healthily work through it, learn from it, and move on. It is believed that the way in which people react or respond to adversity is a very strong indicator of their ability to succeed. So improving your AQ will definitely help to change eating patterns and unzip the fat suit for good!

On the other hand, when something goes wrong for someone with a low AQ, they react in ways that are not aligned with what they really want (sabotaging behaviour).

**Example Scenario:**

A stressful day at work, the boss tells you you've done something wrong. Whether you were right or wrong, it feels as if you are being judged, it feels unfair. Perhaps you decide that what was said is a truth, it confirms to the low AQ mind that you are stupid, unworthy, useless. *(Even if you had done the right thing all along)*.

**Low AQ Scenario:**

**Someone with a low AQ** might drive home seething, furious and frustrated. Perhaps feeling depressed or accepting that they were wrong, even if they were not.

They run the scenario over and over in their mind. If their pattern had been to eat when they felt confronted in this way, they might stop at a store and buy lots of sweets, ice creams and snack foods. They'd start scoffing them in the car and then at home, eat everything till they felt sick, simmering with anger or upset and justifying it in their head.

The inner coach may pipe in every now and then saying, *"Should I really be doing this?"* The inner critic however, continues stimulating the cravings for that old pattern to dominate. The person continues to blame their boss for not understanding them. *"It's the boss's fault that I'm eating this, his/her behaviour made me do this, I deserve this food, and I'll show him/her"*. *Alternatively, they then continue to blame themselves for being so stupid, useless or hopeless.*

On the other hand, if that person in the same scenario had used Control strategies to manage the initial craving or emotional reaction, and they had programmed and rewired their AQ to an increased level of resilience; they would assess the situation and react differently.

**High AQ Scenario**

Someone with a Higher AQ, who had worked on his or her issues, might respond this way instead. Even if they knew the boss had been unfair, they would 'tap' the uncomfortable feelings away. They would calmly drive home contemplating the day. As they passed the old shop where they used to buy ridiculous amounts of food, the inner critic might creep into the mind and say *"Just this once, we deserve a pick me up, we have a reason"*. But the high AQ person now has a stronger inner coach that can reason and see past the craving, emotional need or habit. They react differently now because they know that emotional needs won't be satisfied with food, they now know they need a supportive emotional response. They congratulate themselves and calmly drive past the shop with a smile of triumph. They can't believe they ever wanted to do that to themselves in the past.

At home they eat a normal dinner and assess how to handle the situation with the boss tomorrow. They decide to set up a meeting to discuss what happened. If they were in the right, they would ponder how to calmly stand up for themselves, and, if they were in the wrong, they would calmly ponder how to accept responsibility and apologise.

They go to bed and sleep peacefully, knowing they can sort it easily tomorrow.

**Summary:**

The high AQ person blames no one, they have not taken the issue personally. They assess a situation and ask, *"What can I learn from this?"* The person with a high AQ is in control of their reaction or emotion.

The lower AQ person blames three potential targets: they blame themselves, someone else or the world. They allow the reaction or emotion to control them; they are not in control at all.

If reactive eating patterns such as these have been a concern for you or someone you know in the past, think about how you might respond differently next time you feel confronted, challenged or reactive.

**How might you be able to *respond* to a challenge rather than *react to it*?**

- Would pausing to take a deep belly breath be step 1?
- Could using the 'Power of Three List' be step 2?
- Is using the Control audios and craving buster exercises step 3?
- Would consulting your *inner coach* to '*ask-answer, discuss*' the issue be step 4?
- Will asking the P.I.G. question *'is this satisfying nutritional, habitual or emotional needs'* be step 5?
- Is remembering that emotional needs require an emotional response step 6?
- Would using the Program and Rewire audios daily gradually increase your AQ permanently? Would that help you improve your AQ and become better at dealing with that issue from now on and into the future? Is that a daily step?

**The answer to all of the above questions is a resounding YES!**

Here's a little metaphor that highlights the AQ issue perfectly. After reading this story you may never look at a carrot, an egg, or a coffee bean in the same way. The first time I heard this metaphor, I was in the audience at a therapists' training conference. A colleague read it to the audience as a demonstration of how we can all choose to react differently to adversity, and eventually learn from it. She never told me who the author of the metaphor was, but I honour the author now by sharing it with you.

**When adversity knocks how do you respond? What is your Adversity Quotient?**

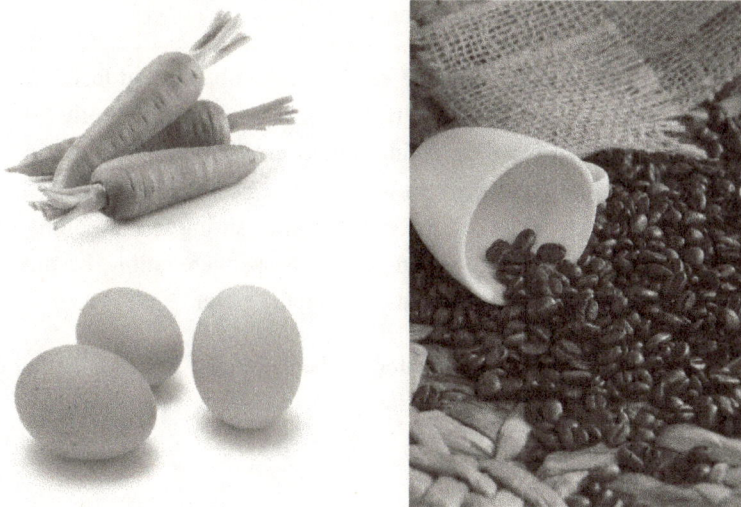

*Author unknown*

A young woman went to her mother and told her how things were so hard for her. She did not know how she was going to make it, and she wanted to give up. She was tired of struggling. It seemed as one problem was solved, a new one arose.

Her mother took her to the kitchen. She filled three pots with water and placed each one on a high fire. Soon the pots came to boil. In the first pot she placed carrots, in the second she placed eggs, and in the last pot she placed ground coffee beans. She let them sit and boil; without saying a word.

In about twenty minutes she turned off the burners. She fished the carrots out and placed them in a bowl. She pulled the eggs out and placed them in a bowl. Then she ladled the coffee out and placed it in a bowl.

Turning to her daughter, she asked, "Tell me what you see."

"Carrots, eggs, and coffee," the daughter replied.

Her mother brought her closer and asked her to feel the carrots. She did and noted that they were soft. The mother then asked the daughter to take an egg and break it. After pulling off the shell, she observed the hard-boiled egg. Finally, the mother asked the daughter to sip the coffee.

The daughter smiled, as she tasted its rich aroma.

The daughter asked, "What does it mean?"

Her mother explained that even though each of these objects had faced the same adversity: 20 minutes of boiling water, they each reacted differently. The carrot went in strong, hard, and unrelenting, however, after being subjected to the boiling water, it softened and became weak. The egg had been fragile, its thin outer shell had protected its liquid interior, but after sitting in the boiling water, its insides became hardened. The ground coffee beans were unique because after they were in the boiling water, they had changed the water.

"Which are you?" she asked her daughter. "When adversity knocks on your door, how do you respond? Are you a carrot, an egg or a coffee bean?

**Exercise:**

Think of this: Which am I? Am I the carrot that seems strong, but with pain and adversity, with complex challenge, do I wilt and become soft and lose my strength? Do I give in to cravings; do I surrender to old habits or patterns? Do I let the emotional pattern or habit control me?

Am I the egg that starts with a malleable heart, but changes with the heat? Did I have a fluid spirit, but after a death, a breakup, a financial hardship, a loss of a job or some other trial, have I become hardened and stiff? Does my shell look the same, but on the inside am I bitter and tough with a stiff spirit and hardened heart? Do I resent challenge; have I stopped caring about my body or myself? Have I allowed reactive, rebellious or self-harming eating patterns to control me?

Or am I like the coffee bean? The bean changed the hot water; it changed the very circumstance that brought the pain. When the water got hot, the bean released its own fragrance and flavour. If you are like the bean, when things are at their worst, you get better. You change the situation around you, rather than let the situation control your reaction or change you. When challenge happens are you at your best? Do you learn from the situation? From today, do you use the strategies that you have learned here to help you become a better person?

Do you face emotional challenges and past patterns with food from a different perspective? Do you use the tools, CPR audios and exercises? Do you understand that when you use these, you are in control of ALL your reactions? Do you change your reaction and do something different this time? Do you then change and inspire the world around you because you now respond to family, people, places and events rather than react to them?

How will you handle adversity, challenging situations or old patterns from today? Will you be a coffee bean? Or will you react using an old pattern and blame the carrot, the egg and the coffee for tempting you then eat them all anyway?

Remember: I can only lead you to water; I can't make you drink it. I can however ask you to trust yourself and me. Please use the CPR audios, please consult your inner coach and please do at least three strategies from any of the solutions in the book, before you respond to new challenges or old patterns!

Taking one step, one day at a time is all you need to do. Choose to use these strategies to disconnect the link between emotions and food. You can take control of your eating patterns from today. I believe in you, it's time for you to start believing in you too.

| Remember your 10 Commitments |
| :---: |
| Rehearse Outfit |
| Audio Daily |
| Weigh Once |
| Stomach chooses |
| Smaller Portions |
| Chew Slowly |
| Push Plate |
| Thirst = Water |
| Wiggle Move |
| Write Progress |

# SEVEN

## Rewire Your Inner Image - I'm Gorgeous: You're Gorgeous

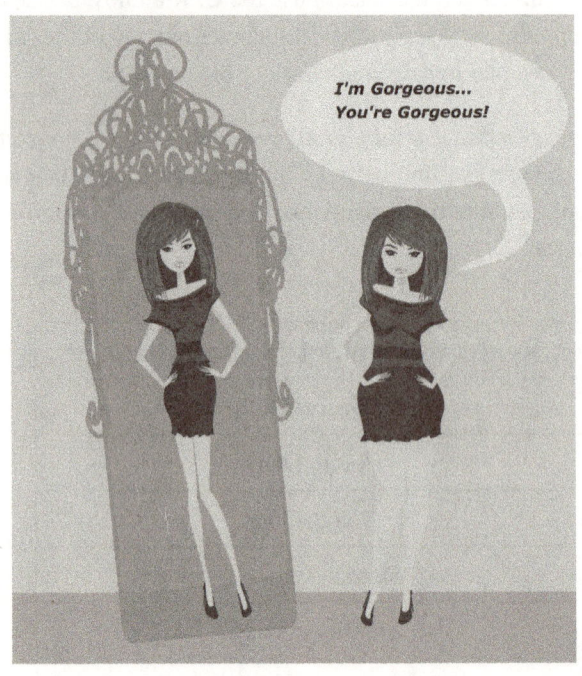

*"It's not who you are that holds you back, it's who you think you're not." Author Unknown*

In order to change unhelpful eating patterns and unzip the fat suit permanently, you also need to build self-confidence. Even if you already have a confident approach to life, it's also important to ensure that you approach your body, your health and your slim and healthy goal with absolute confidence and self-belief too. To do this, it is important to develop strategies to easily deal with and stop:

- The belief, worry or fear about *not being good enough*
- The fear of *what other people think of you*
- The fear of *failure (or success)*
- Self doubt and *doubt in your ability to achieve your slim and healthy goal*
- Procrastination
- Self-sabotaging behaviour

By conquering these issues you will learn how to transform yourself into a confident, healthy, focused and determined person brimming with a calm sense of 'I can'.

*The following three fears are at the core of all of the issues mentioned above. They create lack of confidence, self-doubt, procrastination and sabotaging behaviours. When we let these go, we can create what we want.*

1. Fear of rejection
2. Fear of what other people think of you
3. Fear of making mistakes and failure

To convert self-doubt into self-confidence, procrastination into action and sabotaging behaviour into healthy pro-active behaviour, you need to put into action the strategies provided to let go of these three fears.

Once you have a firm belief that you *can* be slim and healthy permanently, that you *can* change unhelpful habits and reactions, you begin to trust yourself more. You are able to interrupt old unhelpful patterns more easily and willingly.

A comment I hear repeatedly from clients is that as they begin to drop a few kilos, they also begin to feel more confident in many other areas of their life too. All of my CPR audios include confidence and self-esteem suggestions to support the natural development of this process. As you use them, you will automatically notice more of the goodness in your life.

*You will naturally focus more on the positive potential of today and the future, rather than the unhelpful issues of the past.*

Very quickly, you will become aware that weight reduction is not the only benefit you receive when you use the strategies and CPR audios. Life's challenges just seem a little easier within days. You will also notice that you are kinder to yourself, a better friend to you.

As clients naturally grow in confidence and shrink in size, I often hear them say things like *"I can't believe I spent my life worrying about weight." Or "I handle life better now and the extra weight is disappearing anyway."*

In some ways this chapter is the real key. However to make the contents of this chapter work, the steps in the previous chapters and the ones following need to be implemented too. To ensure the change is permanent, you will need to address ALL potential reasons why you originally gained weight, lost confidence, created unhelpful eating patterns, swallowed your emotions or yo-yo dieted in the first place.

When you use my complete package: the 10 Commitments, the CPR audios, the craving control and emotional eating strategies, the mind rehearsal and greedy appetite strategies, then the contents of this chapter begin to happen automatically for you. You simply wake each day, and as your feet touch the floor you know that *'today is a great day to be healthy.'*

The fun exercises and stories I share in this chapter are extra little 'games' to play to help your mind rewire faster. Remember when you do things repeatedly with heightened sensory input (emotions, fun, laughter, play, positive feelings) you rewire your thoughts, habits and emotions more effectively anyway. So why not have fun doing it?

**I mentioned in Chapter 5 that one of my top strategies to rewire unhelpful self-talk was to turn your *inner critic into your inner coach*. Simply ask *"What would my inner coach say or do instead?"* You can also use this technique to rewire and program healthy, confident beliefs and thoughts about your body, mind and your ultimate potential too.**

### 1. Turn your Inner Critic into your Inner Coach

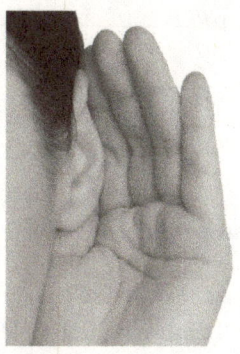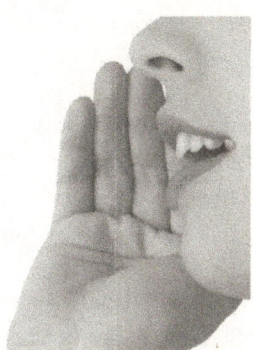

Remember in Chapter 5, I told the story of my 'toxic thinking patterns in London?' Many people do still feel challenged by the ridiculous ramblings of their inner critic. When that niggling (sometimes yelling) voice in the back of the mind goes unchecked, it can often be heard to repeat things like:

- 'I'm too old, I'm too fat, I'm too this or too that...'
- 'I shouldn't, I can't...'
- 'I'm not good enough...'
- 'Others are better...'
- 'What's the point... ?'
- 'I doubt I can...'
- 'What would people think... ?'
- 'I'm useless, hopeless, ridiculous, stupid...'
- I'll never be able to do this.'
- 'What if I fail?'

The list could go on...

If you haven't already begun to address this issue, take a moment to imagine how different it would be if you could transform that unhelpful inner dialogue into support from your inner confidence coach? All it takes is a little vigilance and practice to catch the critic and replace it.

Next time you hear that inner critic...remember the question to ask is:

**'Who's belief is that anyway?** *What would my Inner Coach say or do instead?'*

The National Science Foundation estimates that the human mind produces anywhere from 12,000 to 50,000 thoughts per day, other sources estimate up to 60-70,000. *(Whew I don't envy the person who had to count those thoughts. Whose job was that?)*

It is also often said that out of those 12,000 to 70,000 thoughts each day, about 90% of them are negative. Out of the 90% of the negative or unhelpful thoughts we have, about 90% of those are directed inwardly. Those inwardly directed thoughts are judging, denigrating, accusing, doubting and demeaning of ourselves.

If we look at those statistics conservatively and take the minimum number of thoughts as 12,000 per day, you could potentially have at least 10,800 unhelpful thoughts everyday. Importantly at least 9,720 thoughts would be negative, self-doubting or judgemental thoughts about you! Whew! I'm exhausted just thinking about that!

- Do you ever catch yourself dwelling on old issues, grievances of the past?
- Do you mull over mistakes, beating yourself up because you 'should have done better'?
- Do you have worrying thoughts about loved ones, the future, or the past?
- Do you do judgement thoughts about yourself or others? *"I look too fat in this" or "I'm useless at that".*
- Do you have fear or anxious thoughts about your health or the health of someone you love?
- Do you have doubting thoughts? "I'll never make it" or "Even if I lose the weight, I'll put it back on"

These, and many other thoughts like them, are simply variations on the theme that reinforces self-doubt, procrastination and sabotaging behaviour.

If your mind is busy with unhelpful worrying, judgemental, critical and useless thoughts, it's no wonder that you can't stay focused or motivated to do the things you really want to do for your health.

Remember: Be vigilant about your thoughts. You don't have to be perfect, simply vigilant. If the occasional inner critic thought slips through, then be amused by the lie instead of believing it as truth. Recognise you can change the critical thought into an *inner coach* thought instead.

## Fun Exercise 1:

Commit to catching and changing at least 20% of your inner critic thinking to inner coach thinking for the next 24 hours. Make it a game – you may be amused at how many thoughts there are to change.

Do the same every day for a week. Be on the lookout for the critic and ready with the coach more often.

## 10 Tips & Strategies for Inner Confidence:

1.  If you become aware of Inner Critic thinking about your body or your size and shape, then swap it instantly for Confidence Coach support
2.  Do the things you are afraid of anyway. Ask yourself: *"What's the worst that can happen?"*
3.  You can't grow if you don't learn from mistakes! Decide that the fear of making mistakes *(having to be right)* is not as important as the desire to achieve what you want.
4.  Do one thing differently each week. Step out of your comfort zone and change one eating pattern weekly. *(This can also interrupt your body's patterns too, so it doesn't fall into a habit of plateauing as you move toward your ideal weight, shape and size)*
5.  Use mind rehearsal. Rehearse all positive outcomes, see and feel your success with all of your senses as if it's real now *(Remember the mind doesn't know the difference between real and imagined)*
6.  Do your belief audit regularly *(Use the control tapping exercises on unhelpful beliefs to let them go)*
7.  Be on alert for the alarm phrases: I can't/I shouldn't and change it to 'I can...I do'
8.  Write a list of your good points and read them to yourself every day *(review this list daily and add to it as you go)*
9.  Read your 'I AM' list daily, add to it as you go
10. If these symptoms persist, seek help from a professional. (info@thepotentialist.com )

---

*"It took me a long time not to judge myself through someone else's eyes."* Sally Field

---

## Fun Exercise 2:

## 10 things I like about my body and myself

Write a letter to your body and list the ten things you like about it. Often you become used to focusing on the 'bad' bits and forget that there are bits you do like. Even those with a very poor body image can usually find a few things they do like about themselves, with a little prompting.

We are so used to only focusing on the negative because we have been pro-grammed this way. Even very early at school, I personally remember comparing my body and myself negatively to other kids in my class. It is human nature to want to be like others.

By writing your '10 Things I Like About My Body & Myself List', reading and re-assessing it regularly *(like I suggest you do with your 'I AM' list),* you can monitor your progress. You will recognise as your brain rewires with positive thinking habits, that you notice more positive aspects about your body, and start to instinctually like more about yourself every day.

## 10 Things I Like About My Body and Myself

| | |
|---|---|
| 1 | |
| 2 | |
| 3 | |
| 4 | |
| 5 | |
| 6 | |
| 7 | |
| 8 | |
| 9 | |
| 10 | |

**Have a love affair with your body**

## Accepting Compliments

One of the first ways to start accepting your body more, is to accept compliments more. Too often I hear people justifying the compliments they receive and therefore rejecting them. It is a proud moment when a client recognises the importance of receiving compliments and simply says, 'thank you' when they receive one.

Every time you reject something nice that someone says about you or to you, you are rejecting not only the compliment and your body; you are also rejecting the other person's opinion. You invalidate them. One key to help rewire your inner image and feel more confident is to *hear* a compliment and *accept* it with ease and grace. By acknowledging it, you will eventually learn how to believe it too.

When people are particularly challenged by compliments it shows that they are challenged to accept some part of themselves. When this is the case, I often play a compliments game. This game can be played in small groups or as pairs. If it's pairs, each person takes turns being the compliment giver and then the receiver. The compliment receiver must always accept and acknowledge the compliment using the same technique as the group game, which I will explain now.

## How It works:

One person is chosen to receive compliments. *(Everyone gets a chance to be the receiver before the game is over).* One at a time people give a compliment to the nominated receiver while everyone listens.

Once a compliment has been given, the receiver of the compliment is to receive it appropriately. *(Whether they believe it or not yet, remember we are rewiring the brain).* To make it easier, I offer an example:

## Step one: Compliment giver gives compliment:

The first compliment giver starts by saying to the nominated receiver something like *"Julie, I admire the way your eyes sparkle, you make me feel happy when you smile"*

## Step two: Receiver receives compliment appropriately

Julie responds by saying out loud: "*Thank you* for saying my eyes sparkle and that I make you feel happy when I smile." (First response is always simply *thank you*).

## Step three: Receiver Accepts and acknowledges compliment

Then Julie repeats: "*I **do** have eyes that sparkle and I **do** have a smile that makes people feel happy.*"

Then the next person in the circle would share a genuine compliment about Julie, she would have to respond to that compliment using the same process.

This would continue until everyone in the group had given Julie a compliment. Then, she would repeat all the compliments until she could say them without embarrassment or rejection.

After this, everyone would take his or her turn at being the compliment receiver. The process would continue until everyone had experienced being the receiver.

The difficulty some people have with repeating the compliments back or accepting them as their own still astounds me. I find with the compliments game, it challenges people to accept and to allow goodness in. It challenges them to stop rejecting themselves and others.

By practicing receiving compliments, you will find it is more natural to recognise compliments that you may not have even heard before. When people have lots of unhelpful inner self-talk, their inner critic blocks compliments. That little voice in their head usually responds to compliments with: "*No I'm not*" or "*This old thing...*" or "*Hmm you don't know me very well, do you*".

**Fun Compliments Exercise:** if you have a few close friends that you feel comfortable with, try playing the compliments game. See how comfortable you really are to hear the good stuff about you. Keep playing regularly, until it feels more comfortable.

## Fun Exercise 3:

**Remember step two** in the compliments game is simply to start your response to a compliment with 'thank you'. The same goes for compliments that you receive in everyday life during general conversation. Many people find ways to justify or deny compliments. *"You've got to be kidding, I look like a train wreck today"* or *"This old thing, had it for years"* or *"It was nothing, forget it"*.

What about simply saying *"thank you"* to every compliment you receive this week? Give it a go, and be amused if you hear yourself or others trying to justify their compliments too. Do this exercise all week, I bet you notice a difference by the end of the week.

## Acknowledging the Gold Within You

In chapter 1 of Eckhart Tolle's book "The Power of Now" he opens with a parable about a beggar asking strangers for spare change, while he is sitting on a box that he had never opened. When he did finally open it, Eckhart Tolle says, *"... he saw that the box was filled with gold."* In explanation of this parable, Eckhart suggests, *"I am the stranger that has nothing to give you and who is telling you to look inside. Not in any box, as in the parable, but somewhere even closer: look inside yourself."*

The validation, the compliments, the recognition and love we sometimes seek from others, from our wealth, our career and our family or a friend, is often hollow when we do receive it. If we have become too focused on unhelpful or toxic inner critic thoughts, we often disregard or doubt the compliments and validation we do receive. Sometimes we don't even hear them being offered.

Self-acceptance and self-love, your self-worth and confidence, is the only sustainable 'gold' you need. The validation or recognition you often seek from others actually needs to come from within you first. Once you start looking for, and listening to the potential of the gold within you, you begin to feel more of it and then it flows to you from the outside world too. (This happens because you are able to hear and see more of the goodness outside of you too; you start to let it in).

When people have felt empty inside for long periods, they tend to look to the outside world and only see validation of their emptiness. Even when others are offering us compliments and acknowledgement, we can be numb to everything except how bad we are, or how useless we feel. We don't often see or feel the goodness (gold) being offered. If we haven't acknowledged our own goodness within, we tend to reflect our unworthiness and reject compliments and positivity being offered to us anyway.

We tend to 'need' more, and feel 'blame' if our life, or others do not provide what we want. We can justify our unworthiness, sometimes reveling in the emptiness we think we see outside ourselves. *"See I was right"* we say to ourselves. *"Nobody loves me, I was right all along. I am not worth loving anyway."*

Yet we continue wishing and hoping and wanting. Perhaps it is simply time to get off your box and open the lid. To see more of the gold within you!

**Exercise: think about these questions**

1. What *gold* is within you that you haven't acknowledged yet?
2. What emptiness needs to be rewired for the *goodness* in you to be nurtured and noticed?
3. What *gold* have you begun to notice about yourself as you've progressed so far on this journey to unzip the fat suit and rewire your mind to create healthier eating patterns?
4. What *goodness* have you begun to notice in the world around you that you hadn't noticed before?
5. What *gold* do you hope is yet to be found within?
6. Are you willing to look in the mirror to find that *goodness*?

## I'm Gorgeous: You're Gorgeous

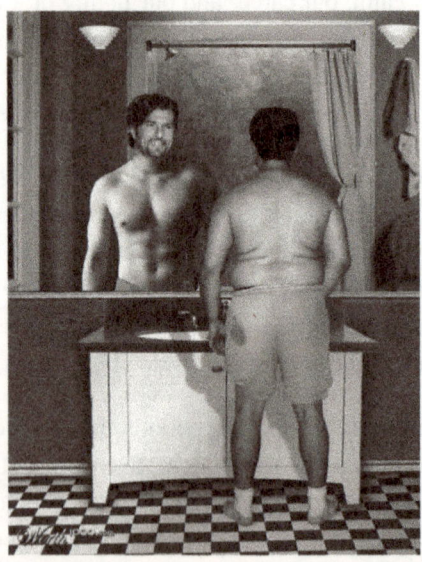

Another exercise I ask clients to do *(and I do this myself every day)* is mirror work.

You may or may not have heard of mirror work before, it is recommended by many self-help and empowerment authors worldwide.

The mirror work that I do is very specific to helping you discover the 'gold' within you. It's my *'I'm Gorgeous; You're Gorgeous'* exercise

(For all the gorgeous guys out there if you are uncomfortable using the word 'gorgeous', simply replace it with hunky, sexy or handsome, whatever word works for you. Personally, I think you're all gorgeous too).

## This is how it works:

Step 1: Stand in front of the mirror in the morning and again, last thing at night

Step 2: Take a deep breath, and no matter how silly or uncomfortable you feel at first, commit to looking yourself in the eye, pointing both hands to your physical body as you say: '*I'm Gorgeous*' with as much energy as you can muster

Step 3: Then point with both hands to your reflection in the mirror and say: *"You're Gorgeous"* with even more energy.

Repeat this three times at least once or twice per day.

Remember, your brain learns faster when you experience heightened sensations and feelings, and of course repetition, so the more you do this and the more energy you put into it, the faster your brain will learn. Once you start doing this, you will begin to notice the goodness in you more, and you'll start to believe how gorgeous, handsome, sexy and hunky you really are!

*(Do this often enough and eventually you'll end up doing it silently in your mind when you catch a glimpse of your reflection in a shop window, or at your reflection in the mirror when you wash your hands)*

## Fun Exercise 4:

Do the *"I'm Gorgeous: You're Gorgeous"* game everyday till it no longer feels uncomfortable or silly. Do it till it feels fun and even normal. Make it a great habit.

Remember, when rewiring your brain with a new behaviour, belief or habit; there are sometimes 'uncomfortable' feelings that can occur as a result of the new electrical circuitry in your brain. It is often even a physical sensation as your brain rewires new thought patterns. You might remember when you learned to drive a car? Or started a new job with new tasks? Or learned something new, like a musical instrument or a language, a new sport? At first, there were uncomfortable squirmy feelings. Often as we learn there are thoughts that say 'I'm no good at this' or 'this is ridiculous, there's no point', 'this is too hard'.

Eventually, when you persisted with whatever you were learning, it became easy for you. For those of us who have been driving a car for years, we don't even have to think about how much pressure to put on the brakes in order to pull up at a traffic light or a stop sign, do we? Our brain has done this so often, it runs on automatic pilot.

So when practicing these exercises, the *'Compliments Game'*, the *'10 Things I Like about Myself and My Body'* game and the *'I'm Gorgeous: You're Gorgeous'* game, it's important to continue doing them until they feel comfortable. This is the best sign, because this means you have programmed and rewired new, more positive neural pathways that bring you closer to where you want to be. Closer to the confidence you need to help you change your eating patterns and unzip the fat suit for good!

## The $20.00 Note
### *Author Unknown*

This little story has been bandied about in therapeutic circles for years. I do not unfortunately know the origins, however the importance of its meaning is very clear and very relevant to this chapter. If anyone is aware of its origins please let me know so that I can reference it properly next time.

A well-known presenter stood in front of a large audience and held up a $20 note. He said *'Who would like this $20 note?'* Lots of people put their hands up. Over the next few minutes he pulled out a pair of scissors and snipped the corners off the note, then he crumpled it, dropped it, kicked it, stood on it and ground it into the floor. He then asked *'Who still wants it?'* More hands went up.

The presenter then proceeded to tell the audience that they had learned a valuable lesson. No matter what he had done to the $20, people still saw its value, its value never decreased, and it constantly remained worth $20.

Many times throughout life we are chopped, cut, dropped, crumpled, stood on, climbed over, ground into the dirt and treated like crap by circumstances, people, and events. The decisions we make, or the actions or inactions of others or ourselves, can often leave us feeling broken. Many times we feel as though we are worthless, useless and hopeless. But no matter what has actually happened, or not happened, or will happen, or could happen, you never lose your value at all.

Dirty or clean, crumpled or creased, beaten or hurt, fat or thin, healthy or sick, abandoned or rejected, abused or loved, you are priceless. You always remain worthy. You were born worthy, and so shall you remain, no matter what does or does not happen.

The worth of our lives comes not from what we do, or who we know, or what we earn or what we have, but, from who we are.

**Remind yourself often of this important fact:**

You are worthy! You are worthy of love, worthy of health, worthy of strength, worthy of joy, worthy of compliments, worthy of beauty, worthy of wealth, worthy of life, worthy of a voice and especially worthy of hugs.

No matter what does or does not happen in life... No matter who does what to who... your value always remains the same. You are always worthy of health and love. You were not born *with* self-doubt; you learned how to *do* self-doubt.

You were born a divine, loving child worthy of love, and you remain a divine loving person, worthy of love, always. So look in that mirror and say: "I am gorgeous, handsome, hunky and sexy!"

## Two Self Confidence audios

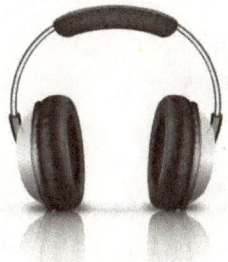

Remember if you haven't already started using my Program and Rewire audios for confidence and self-esteem do so, from today. I have also provided a cardio version of each of these audios, so that you can use them while you wiggle and move your body too.

## Rewire Confidence and Self Esteem Audio:

Use this audio regularly throughout the day, and while walking or exercising to support the change process. It's only a few minutes long so repetition is the key.

The types of suggestions to expect within this audio are below.

## Rewire for Confidence

I am worthy of health
I am worthy of love
I am worthy of prosperity
I am worthy of greatness

I have permission to be healthy
I have permission to love and be loved
I have permission to be prosperous
I have permission to be great

I am worthy of respect
I am worthy of joy
I am worthy of confidence
I am worthy of kindness

I treat myself with respect
I treat myself with joy
I treat myself with confidence
I treat myself with kindness

I am worthy of happiness
I am worthy of compassion
I am worthy of love
I am worthy of talents and abilities

I experience happiness
I experience compassion
I experience love
I experience my talents and abilities

I am worthy of peace
I am worthy of wisdom
I am worthy of friendship
I am worthy of strength

I allow peace in
I allow wisdom in
I allow friendship in
I allow strength in

I am worthy of prosperity
I am worthy of knowledge
I am worthy of life
I am worthy of forgiveness

I give myself prosperity
I give myself knowledge
I give myself life
I give myself forgiveness

I am worthy of motivation
I am worthy of success
I am worthy of freedom
I am worthy of love

I create motivation
I create success
I create freedom
I create love

I am worthy of positive energy
I am worthy of peaceful stillness
I am worthy of receiving help
I am worthy of divine protection

I am positively energised
I am peacefully still
I am able to receive help
I am divinely protected

I am worthy
I honour myself and my talents and abilities
I forgive myself
I like and love who I am
I am worthy
I feel good

◆

This is a prayer I wrote to my body many years ago. I did this when I finally realised how unkind I had been to it with my inner critic thoughts and actions. This prayer was one of the steps I used to start the journey to accept and love my body and myself, to find the *gold* and the goodness within me.

When you feel ready, you may wish to write your own prayer to your body, perhaps you might write it in your progress journal, in Chapter 14.

## Prayer to my body
### *By Maggie Wilde*

Dear Body,

I am sorry that I have been unkind; I have treated you like an enemy sometimes, instead of as a friend. If I am not present in you, accepting of you, and kind to you, you start to deteriorate, age and become diseased and eventually you will die. I know I have not been present for you very often, and I am truly sorry dear body.

You exist to protect me. You have life when I am present in you. All these years, I did not see that. I treated you as though you were my slave, and not my friend or my protector.

If I did recognise you as my friend dear body:

I would have loved you, instead of hated you,

I would have accepted you, instead of rejected you.

I would have had fun with you, instead of shut you down.

I would have let you play sometimes, instead of making you work all day.

I would have let you live with joy.

There are not many times dear body, that I have allowed you to feel alive. Sometimes you had to scream at me so that I would listen. And even then I often did not. And I am sorry, so very sorry that I did not hear you dear body, until now.

I love you and I accept you

I am grateful for every cell in you, the patience you have shown me even when my kindness was absent. You struggled along with a strength that is truly miraculous and until now, I hardly ever noticed that you were miraculous at all.

So dear body, thank you. I am truly grateful to you. From the top of my head down. To every cell every muscle every sinew of this body, I am grateful, I choose to direct my awareness and kindness back to this body, to listen, acknowledge, hear this body more.

I thank you. I am not just my mind, I am not just my body, I am the essence that has been gifted with two of the most amazing strengths. A mind that is *so strong* and a body that *is so strong,* and I acknowledge that now.

Thank you mind, thank you body.

You are my friend dear body, I love you

You are my friend dear body, I accept you

**You are my friend dear body, I choose to have fun with you**

I choose to be kind to you, I choose to let you play, and I accept you, more every day.

| Remember your 10 Commitments |
|:---:|
| Rehearse Outfit |
| Audio Daily |
| Weigh Once |
| Stomach chooses |
| Smaller Portions |
| Chew Slowly |
| Push Plate |
| Thirst = Water |
| Wiggle Move |
| Write Progress |

# EIGHT

## Rewire Digestion - Choose How to Chew

**Why Chewing More Slowly and More Often, Helps Makes You Slim**

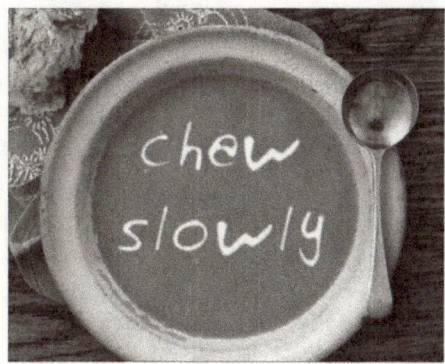

In Chapter 2, I outlined the 10 Commitments that help you rewire unhelpful patterns and unzip the fat suit permanently. I briefly discussed that chewing more slowly was one of those important commitments, and I will delve a little deeper into the importance of that topic in this chapter.

A team of researchers from Iowa State University studied students while they were eating. Assistant Professor of Food Science and Human Nutrition, James Hollis reported their findings at the Experimental Biology Conference held in California in April 2012. (http://archive.news.iastate.edu/news/2012/apr/chewing)

Students in the study were given pizza, they were told to chew every time a metronome clicked. 50% of the students had to chew 15 times to the metronome before swallowing, and the other half had to chew 40 times in unison with the metronome before swallowing.

**The student's appetites were monitored, and those who chewed more, ate less food and their hunger levels reduced. They literally consumed fewer calories.**

Importantly, the students' blood levels were monitored during the research and those who chewed more had *an increase in a hormone called CCK*. This hormone is related to the sensation of *fullness and satisfaction*. For the students who chewed more, there was also a *reduction in another hormone called 'ghrelin'*; ghrelin is a hormone involved in stimulating appetite.

This meant that the students who chewed more:

- Ate less *and*
- Had a greater sense of satisfaction
- They literally had smaller appetites

This is one of the very important reasons to practice chewing more often and more slowly. By chewing slowly and more often, you will want less food and feel more satisfied than before. Less food, equals less kilojoules. Hmm, are you getting the simplicity of that?

James Hollis was reported to say that, *"When people chewed the pizza 40 times before swallowing, there was a reduction in hunger, preoccupation with food and their desire to eat"*.

Now, chewing 40 times per mouthful for fibrous foods such as meats or crunchy vegetables and salads may be reasonably easy to achieve, however, you might find chewing mashed potato or soup 40 times quite challenging. Remember it is the mindful, conscious way you approach chewing that is the key here, *not the exact number* of chews.

Chewing 40 times is the optimal scientific level. Be aware of the importance of chewing slowly and mindfully, and work up to the optimal levels where you can. The key is simply to practice a mindful approach to eating and gradually add a few chews to each mouthful at first.

Secondly, when you eat as though you are competing in a contest, shovelling the next mouthful in before you have even swallowed the one before; you miss out on a deeper appreciation of the flavours and textures of food. When people are in the habit of 'inhaling' food, or gulping it down, eating tends to become habitual or 'a way to fill the emptiness', rather than a joyful experience.

When food is appreciated, when the flavours and textures of each mouthful are contemplated with pleasure, then it helps you enjoy the quality of the food, not just the quantity of it. Feeling satisfied is an important success component of permanent weight-reduction and changing eating habits. The top two reasons dieters say they have given up on diets in the past highlights why this is an important issue to address:

## Top 2 Reasons People Give Up on Diets

1. Hunger (I don't feel satisfied – I haven't had enough)
2. Missing out on food they enjoy (I don't feel satisfied – why can't I have what I want?)

So if chewing more often and more slowly increases your satisfaction levels, without increasing the quantity of kilojoules you ingest, it is definitely a very beneficial strategy to practice.

In Commitment 4, Chapter 2, I stressed that choosing how to chew was very important in relation to creating a healthy digestive system too. When our digestive system functions optimally, reducing weight is easier and faster.

> Chewing is directly related to the enzymes you need to digest your food. Saliva contains its *own digestive enzymes*. The slower and longer you *chew*, the more time these enzymes have to start processing your food while it is still in your mouth. The chewing stimulates enzyme production in the stomach too. A signal is sent from the brain to the stomach when you chew telling the stomach that it should produce more digestive enzymes in preparation for the food that is about to be swallowed.

> According to Mireille Guiliano, the author of *"French Women Don't Get Fat"*, it takes 20 minutes for the brain to interpret and communicate the satisfied feeling. This makes it even more imperative to chew slowly and more often. The longer you take to eat your smaller portions, the more your stomach and brain register satisfaction. It helps you realise that you're full.

Chewing food well stimulates the gastric juices and enzymes in the stomach to effectively digest the food. The stomach juices and enzymes process food until it's a paste called chyme. Once this happens it can then move through into the small intestine. This takes a lot of energy to do, which is why we can feel lethargic after

163

eating a big meal (remember *food coma*?). Up to 70% of the body's energy is diverted to process food.

If food reaches your stomach and is still in large un-chewed chunks, digestion becomes exhausting for your body and takes longer to do. If food is chewed well, then less energy is needed for digestion, and your body can use that energy elsewhere.

Chewing well also decreases the chance that food will sit undigested, fermenting in your stomach.

**Fermentation = gas = flatulence = bloating = the other 'f' word … fart!**

Now, that's something we all want to avoid!

As a bonus for our health also, chewing slower and more often stimulates glands in front of the ears that are part of our immune system. So stimulating these glands by chewing more, can give your immune system a boost too. Your body is designed so cleverly don't you think?

I've already established that by chewing slowly, you give the body and stomach time to catch up with how satisfied you feel. You literally give your stomach time to recognise it's fuller far sooner than before. As a result of this, you begin to want less food. Voila! Smaller portions, which is another one of our Commitments!

Make the commitment to yourself that you will begin to enjoy every mouthful more and saviour the food. Enjoy the texture of the food, chew more times and enjoy the flavours and smells as you chew. Relax as you eat, think and feel positively about the food you are eating and of course, do it more slowly.

Take smaller bites too. Remember when you do this; you become aware that there is much more pleasure in the eating process, not just the quantity of food. It helps shift the focus from quantity to quality and it helps shift the body from the stressed state to the relaxed state. When this happens, we reach our weight and size goal faster.

**In summary so far**

- Research shows chewing up to 40 times is helpful to satisfaction levels and consuming less kilojoules
- Simply practice being more mindful of how many times you chew and the pace you chew. Don't get too hung up on the exact number, just add a few chews to each mouthful at first, as you build to optimal levels

- If you have been an 'inhaler' of food, (eating as though you are in a race) then aim at first for 15 to 30 chews and then see how you go from there
- Take more time to eat your meal (20 minutes approx). This creates more satisfaction levels so the need to 'nibble' on something else after a meal diminishes. It also helps our body relax and we reach our goals faster
- Put your cutlery down between mouthfuls. Or if you are eating finger food or a sandwich, put the food down between each mouthful and focus on the textures, smells and flavours of the food as you chew
- Pause between mouthfuls after you have swallowed to consult your stomach for the satisfied feeling before taking another mouthful
- Consult your inner coach and ask the *P.I.G. question: "Is this mouthful satisfying nutritional, habitual or my emotional needs?"*
- If you feel a heavy fullness you have already overeaten. This causes more stress on the digestive system and therefore affects other systems in the body too
- Check-in for a comfortable or satisfied sensation or feeling, an inner knowing that says 'enough is enough'

## Television, Busy-ness and Food

It is also important that you do not eat in front of the television, while reading, distracted by other things or working. When you do this you will be less conscious of what you are eating or the way you are chewing. Remember, your mind does not know the difference between real and imagined, so it needs to 'see' the food disappearing in front of you to understand and register that you've eaten. To create that satisfied comfortable feeling, it helps to look at your plate or the food you are eating.

If you are watching television, then your mind will believe that whatever is happening on the screen in front of you, is happening in your lounge room. So if there is something stressful, highly emotional or distracting on the television, then your mind will respond by producing stress hormones to deal with the situation as if it is real. If it is stressful or upsetting, your mind will have shifted you into the fight, flight or freeze (FFF) response and therefore, it will have disrupted digestion (refer to the chart following).

So take the time to sit down and focus on the food in front of you. Chew up to 40 times for each mouthful. Pause after each mouthful, check-in for the comfortable, satisfied feeling and recognise when 'enough is enough' then push the plate away.

## The Link Between Chewing, Digestion and Stress

The connection between stress and chewing and the role that this plays in our digestive process is important to address too.

| Your Autonomic Nervous System is made up of two parts | |
| --- | --- |
| **The Sympathetic Nervous System *(SNS)*** <br><br> **The Fight, Flight or Freeze (FFF) Response** <br><br> In FFF you have: <br><br> • Increased Heart Rate <br> • Increased Adrenalin & Cortisol levels <br> • Increased energy / blood sent to limbs in order to run or fight <br> • Increased blood pressure <br> • Reduced capacity for digestion <br><br> When you chew fast and inhale food <br><br> • Your body is constantly in this state of tension FFF <br> • Digestion is affected and nutrients cannot be absorbed appropriately <br> • Energy that is normally used to digest food is diverted to limbs or other systems in the body to prepare you to run, freeze or fight <br> • If you chew too fast as if you are in a race you create the stress FFF response. | **Parasympathetic Nervous System *(PNS)*** <br><br> **This is the Rest and Digest (R/D) Response** <br><br> In R/D you have: <br><br> • Healthy working digestive system <br> • Healthy, regular waste elimination <br> • A calmer outlook in the body and mind <br> • Calmer thoughts <br> • Your body heals <br> • Your circulation / blood pressure returns to normal <br> • Your body, organs, muscles relax and regenerate <br><br> **Very importantly** <br><br> Each time you are in this relaxed, R/D state, you can process and eliminate foods far more easily. You absorb the nutrients and eliminate the waste more easily because you activate more digestive enzymes. |

*(continued)*

166

| The Sympathetic Nervous System *(SNS)* | Parasympathetic Nervous System *(PNS)* |
|---|---|
| • When you eat when you are already stressed, if you eat on the run or spend too much time in this stress mode, your digestive system can be affected long term. You will find it more difficult to lose weight / relax / eliminate waste and toxins from the body<br>• When you eat while distracted or busy, your body is in *FFF.* Digestion is difficult and the nutrients cannot be absorbed appropriately. (Hence people can develop reflux, irritable bowel syndrome (IBS), ulcerative colitis or leaky gut amongst so many other things<br>• When you regularly eat in a stressed way the body will store excess fat to protect the organs, muscles and fibres from aging as a result of the stress. It will simply become more challenging to reduce weight and change eating patterns | Each time you use CPR audios and other strategies in this book you activate digestion and your body eliminates waste more easily. When you eat or chew in a relaxed way you automatically shift from *the SNS to the PNS. When this happens unzipping the fat suit and changing patterns* becomes easier.<br><br>Being in the *PNS* helps you unzip the fat suit, feel calmer, de-stress, heal and feel peaceful. It lengthens your life and makes you a happier person to be around too.<br><br>When people with stress related health issues such as reflux, IBS, ulcerative colitis or leaky gut begin to eat in a more relaxed way and use the CPR audios, they access the PNS and R/D allows their symptoms to ease too. |

## Re-activating The Stomach's Intelligence

Many overweight clients have come into my office saying: "*I don't ever feel hungry*" or "*I can't tell if I'm full or not, I don't feel anything until I am bulging and uncomfortable*".

One of the keys to reactivating your stomach's natural intelligence for sensing hunger and fullness is the commitment you make to chewing more slowly and eating mindfully.

You were born with an original internal intelligence system that registered this sensation of fullness and hunger, and you can relearn, reactivate and rewire your thinking to hear it, feel it and sense it again. As a baby, you instinctually pushed the bottle or the breast away when you were full. As a toddler if you had had enough, you pushed the plate away.

You can learn to do this again by pausing after you swallow each mouthful, checking in with your brain and stomach to listen out for what is needed. By doing this, you can re-activate that innate intelligence and recognise again when enough is enough. To help you do this, the CPR audios have suggestions woven into them to help reprogram this ability. Before long, you will have reactivated your original weight control mechanism, the innate intelligence to sense genuine hunger and fullness. You will once again be motivated to respond to it by pushing the food away, like you did as a toddler and baby.

This is all the more reason to listen to the CPR audios regularly.

Remember between mouthfuls, put your cutlery or food down, pause and consult your inner coach to ask your P.I.G. question: *"Is this mouthful satisfying nutritional, habitual or my emotional needs?"* Then consult your stomach too, does it feel heavy and uncomfortable with what you are eating or the quantity? Or does it feel light and relaxed? These little strategies will surely help you slow the whole eating process down, leading to less consumption and more satisfaction too!

| Remember your 10 Commitments |
|:---:|
| Rehearse Outfit |
| Audio Daily |
| Weigh Once |
| Stomach chooses |
| Smaller Portions |
| Chew Slowly |
| Push Plate |
| Thirst = Water |
| Wiggle Move |
| Write Progress |

# NINE

## Program – Motivation to Move Your Body More

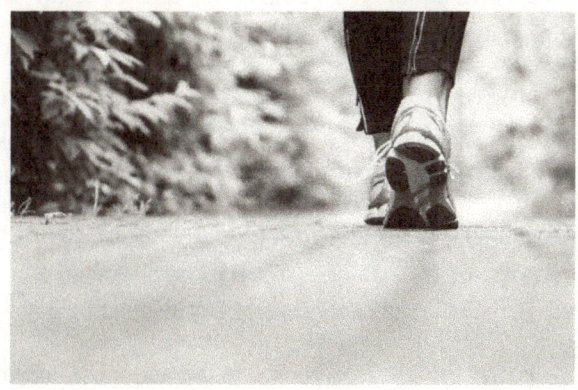

Your body was born to move. You were born eager to wiggle, sit up, crawl then walk. From an early age you wanted to go places, movement meant exploration and play. So guess what? It's time to get moving again!

I need to mention a very specific word now that some people are 'challenged' by. In some people's vocabulary it is a very 'dirty' word and one to be avoided at all costs. In other people's vocabulary it is an exciting word.

### It's the big 'E' word. Exercise!

When dealing with issues of health and weight reduction, one of the most common things that my clients feel challenged by is the topic of exercise. With this in mind, I have devoted this chapter and a couple of CPR audios to this important topic.

Many people know they *should* exercise, they know why they *should* and they make many promises to themselves that they will start *tomorrow*. Then when tomorrow comes they find themselves rolling over in bed with a groan when the alarm goes off. They press snooze while thinking drowsily "Just ten more minutes" or "I'll start tomorrow".

If there are excuses regarding unzipping the fat suit at all, they are more often than not associated with moving the body or exercising. Most of us know what to do, but many of us simply don't do it. Those that don't often feel confused or guilty that they haven't yet found the motivation nor made the commitment to get started. Or they give up within a few weeks or days of starting.

I often wonder how many unused treadmills are in people's garages? I also wonder how many unused gym memberships go wasted around the world? We could probably solve third world famine if we sold all the unused equipment, refunded all the memberships and gave the money to charity.

Remember I'm not perfect; I've been there. I've been the one to roll over and mumble to myself "I'll do it tomorrow". I have lost count of the number of gym memberships I found excuses not to use before I rewired my mind.

If I had a dollar for every time someone said to me "I just don't like exercise" and a dollar for every time I personally said 'I'll walk tomorrow', I would be very prosperous indeed. Perhaps I could solve world famine, just by donating that.

In this chapter, I discuss the excuses people make and ways in which we can overcome them. I will address ways to prioritise moving your body that are in alignment with your desire to be slim and healthy. I discuss my Program audio - *Motivation to Move your Body and Exercise* and the other Control and Rewire audios that help reinforce your ability to rewire your mind to prioritise and look forward to movement every day.

If you already do prioritise movement and enjoy it, these audios will simply help you gain more benefits and enjoy it more. If you don't enjoy it as yet, you will somehow want to soon. It will be easy, you will simply want to do it and there will no longer be an inner conflict or battle about it in your head.

Before I discuss some effective strategies, it is important to understand why many of us find consistent exercise, or even getting off the lounge, challenging. Why some of us have gym memberships going to waste or have cancelled numerous ones we didn't use. Why some of us do roll over and flick the snooze button or curl up our mouth with dislike when the 'E' word is mentioned. Why some of us love it, and why some of us will use every excuse to avoid it.

## Understanding the Role of your Amygdala - your 'Perception Library'

I alluded to this subject earlier in the book, however to understand why some people love exercise and why some don't, we need to get a bit technical about the brain.

This information will help you understand that whatever your attitude to 'exercise' is, it can be reprogrammed and rewired if you choose to do so. Your attitude can be enhanced and even changed, if necessary, by showing you how to stimulate more natural motivation. You can change whatever you need to change, in order to move more and even, dare I say this, enjoy it.

I promise to make this information about your brain as interesting and easy to understand as I can.

Earlier in the book I mentioned the part of your brain called the amygdala. It is a small almond sized gland at the front of the brain and in simplistic terms, one of its roles is a storage library. It stores all your emotional perceptions and interpretations of everything that ever happened or did not happen in your life. It stores your perceptions of every memory you have, including the people and events. As the memory was being stored in one part of your brain, your *'Perception Library'* was also storing and cataloguing your reaction to that memory.

## Why is this important for exercise and movement of the body?

Let's use the scenario below to help understand the importance.

## Exercise Scenario

Let's pretend for a moment you had a physical education (PE) teacher at school or a personal trainer who shouted at you. Someone who said you were hopeless, or they made you feel bad regarding your physical capabilities or sporting prowess.

Perhaps other school students laughed at you during a sporting activity. Perhaps you were made to feel less adequate or clumsier than other students and you were always the last person to be picked for a team sport. Maybe you always dreaded school sports days or swimming carnivals, because you always came last. Or no matter how good you were at sports, you had a friend, brother or sister who was always 'better' than you.

In each of these scenarios, you stored the memories in the cerebrum *(if you were holding your brain in your hand, the cerebrum is the outer surface area of the brain)*

Once these memories were stored, they were stored for life. From then on, every time you're in a situation where you are challenged to do exercise, join a sporting team or participate in sporting activities with friends, then your *'Perception Library', (which catalogues your judgements about those memories)* would respond by calling up the old wounded perception from your past.

Years later, if you decide it's time to get fit and you join a gym, or you make a New Year's resolution to exercise in order to 'lose weight', then it would search for the 'bad' feelings you experienced. It would communicate the uncomfortable perception to the *'Pharmacist'* of your brain.

Remember the *'Pharmacist'* controls your body's production of corticosteroids, (the Neuro-chemicals and stress hormones that create physiological responses to stimuli). Your *'Pharmacist'* determines which Neuro-chemicals should be released in response to the *'Perception Library's'* message. In this example the Neuro-chemicals released determine how you feel, your emotional and physiological response to thinking about exercise, joining the gym or being asked to take part in a team sport with friends.

Depending on what perception was communicated to the *'Pharmacist'*, it will release Neuro-chemicals that will either help you feel motivated (feel good endorphins) or it will release stress hormones that diminish motivation, make you procrastinate, feel uncomfortable, lethargic or disinterested.

If the emotional perception of the old memory was shame, dread or embarrassment, *('I came last', 'I'm so clumsy' or 'I was always picked last')* then that could stimulate an unconscious sensation of fear or upset. You may not consciously remember the past memory or wound from the playground or sporting field, but in the physical world today you interpret this feeling as: "I hate exercise".

Once the *'Pharmacist'* activates the Neuro-chemical in response to the *'Perception Library's'* negative interpretation of the past, today's conclusion would be: I feel absolutely no motivation or desire to do it.

It would be as if you opened the door to the library and the librarian said:

- I'm not the kind of person who enjoys exercise
- I'm not good at sports or exercise
- I'm be so bad at this

- I'll embarrass myself, so why bother
- I won't enjoy this
- There's no point, I'll never follow through
- I'll never win this battle
- I can't be bothered

Unfortunately, when you decide to rewire for slim and healthy, that toxic self-talk, those unhelpful beliefs and decisions you made about yourself back then, cause disinterest, lack of motivation, inability to commit to activity for sustainable periods, procrastination and lack of follow through.

You may not be aware consciously of the interpretation; in fact all you experience today is lack of motivation causing another excuse to pop into your mind. *'I don't have time' or 'I'll do it tomorrow'.*

The emotion or resistance you experience is a reactive response. It's a subconscious, not a conscious one. If you haven't yet learned to rewire that response, then the old programming can be strong enough to override the conscious will to become more active. The battle in your head between the healthy you and the unhealthy you continues.

Only when you reinforce a *new positive 'memory'* over the old one will the motivation change. Remember you can do this because the mind does not know the difference between real and imagined. With regular use of the CPR audios, mind rehearsal *(pretending as if you feel great after exercise)* and repetitively using your progress journal to pre-program a better response to exercise (refer to Chapter 14), you can create those new 'memories' (neural connections).

Once this new 'memory' has been established it will cause the 'Librarian of your *Perception Library'* to communicate a different message to the *'Pharmacist'*. It will now stimulate feel good endorphins creating motivation instead of excuses, enjoyment instead of indifference or rejection.

Here are the steps to programming and rewiring the *'Perception Library'* so that it communicates to your *'Pharmacist'* to release endorphins when you think about moving your body more:

1.  Use Control audios to overcome the feeling of resistance, lethargy or old cellular memories, unhelpful images and feelings about exercise
2.  Repetitively use the Program audio 'Motivation to Move your Body and Exercise'

3.  Repetitively use the Rewire audio – Rewire for Slim and healthy - Unzip the Fat Suit (cardio or relaxation versions)
4.  Repetitively use Mind Rehearsal, imagining 'as if' you have already exercised and feel great. Imagine the feeling after you have already moved your body, how good your body feels and how proud your mind is. Pretend it if you have to at first, you are 'creating' a new 'memory'
5.  Write in your progress journal daily 'as if' you already enjoy exercise. Pretend it if you have to. Perhaps it might help you to remember a time when you did feel proud or motivated about something else, and add that feeling to your mind rehearsal when you think of movement
6.  **Repeat to yourself regularly throughout the day:** *"I'm the kind of person who enjoys moving my body more."*

## An Important Key - Re-assess your Concept of Exercise

As part of the process I used to reprogram my mind for healthy movement of my body, I chose to no longer use the word 'exercise'. I now consider it healthy movement of my body. I choose to move and wiggle my body in ways that help me feel more alive. Ways in which I can have fun. So think outside the box. If you don't like pumping it at a gym, park your car further away from where you need to be and walk more. Sign up for dance lessons or crank up your favourite tunes at home, and dance and wiggle your body more. Find ways to incorporate more 'movement' into your day doing the things you like to do and expand upon the things you normally do.

When we move more – we earn our food, our body then needs the nutrition. Remember the reason we eat is to provide nutrition for the body to live, so ask before every meal:

*"Have I moved my body enough today that it now needs the nutrition in this food?"*

Hmm… Smaller portions – chew slowly and move more – it could all be that simple

## Top Tips You Need to Know To Earn Your Food

*   Plan an activity before every meal or straight after it
*   Only give your body the fuel and nutrition it needs to be healthy (smaller portions)
*   Make choices about food with your stomach, not with your mouth or head
*   Remember to ask your Inner Coach the P.I.G question: *Is this mouthful satisfying nutritional, habitual or my emotional needs?*

Note to Self: Practice self-acceptance; never compare yourself when you move your body to others in any way. There are only two reasons we ever do that.

1.  The first reason is to help you feel better by justifying that they seem worse than you (This is not compassionate to them)
2.  The second reason is to make you feel worse (punish you) because they seem better than you. (This is not compassionate to you)

Either way, comparison doesn't help, it hinders your progress and it is energy that could be better spent reminding yourself about the positive things, the helpful things you did today.

**Mind Rehearse** your ideal weight, shape and size many times throughout every day. Imagine wearing your goal outfit, working out or walking, dancing having active fun. See it, feel it, pretend it is already so. Remember you know by now that your mind won't know the difference and you'll get there faster (and with more joy).

**Use the 10 Commitments daily** and **the CPR audios** and have fun.

Eliminate unhelpful thoughts, beliefs, attitudes and emotions. Recognise excuses and have a giggle at your persistence, then let it go and move on. Key is … *move* on!

Know your strengths and use them to your advantage. Identify your challenges and be ready to work on them or ask for help to move through them.

## The 12 Steps to Healthy Eating and Perfect Athleticism

In Chapter 13, I introduce you to Sharny and Julius Kieser. They are fitness experts who are taking the fitness and health industries by storm. Their 12-step fitness approach for healthy eating and perfect athleticism is provided in detail in that chapter, so I won't go into detail here.

For now, all you need to be aware of is that steps 1 through 5 of their 12-step process are particularly significant for this chapter on moving the body. In short, Sharny and Julius' perspective on fitness and weight reduction is that you are already an athlete; the only issue is that you currently have a winter coat of fat on.

In my terms, it's simply time to unzip the fat suit so that you can discover your inner athlete… yeah!

When Michelangelo created his sculptured masterpiece David, he was reportedly asked questions like: *"How did you carve such a perfect David out of one piece of marble?"* He allegedly replied along these lines: *"David was already in the marble, I simply chipped away the excess."*

In my opinion, Sharny and Julius' perspective is based on a similar principle. The perfect specimen that is you, *is already* an athlete, that athlete is already inside you. It's simply time to chip away the excess winter coat, and unhelpful patterns, to reveal the perfect specimen and athlete within.

You can read Sharny and Julius' full process in Chapter 13. I send a big thank you to them for their valuable input. Their message is quite simple: you were born an athlete, unhelpful behaviours and habits created a winter coat, and now it's time to take responsibility to take it off.

**Or as I would say: Unzip the fat suit for good to discover the slim and healthy you!**

## Time Management – Is there Room for Exercise?

This little story offers an interesting perspective on prioritising life and creating time for the things that really matter - our health and the things we need to do to create that.

When things in your life seem almost too much to handle, when 24 hours in a day are not enough, remember this metaphor.

### The Mayonnaise Jar and the 2 Glasses of Wine...
#### *Author unknown*

A professor stood before his philosophy class with a large empty mayonnaise jar and filled it with golf balls. He then asked the students if the jar was full. They agreed that it was.

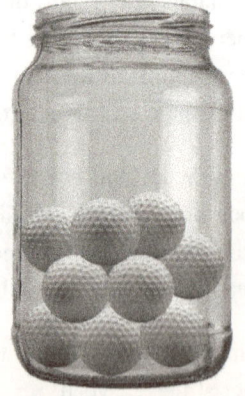

He then poured pebbles into the jar and shook it till the pebbles filled the space between the golf balls. He asked the students again if the jar was full, and they agreed it was.

The professor then poured sand into the jar. The sand filled the space between the pebbles and golf balls. He asked again if the jar was full. The students responded with a unanimous 'Yes'.

He poured two glasses of wine into the jar, effectively filling the empty space between the sand.

"Now" said the professor, as the laughter subsided, "I want you to recognise that this jar represents your life. The golf balls are the important things: your family, your children, your health, your physical fitness and your friends. They represent your passions, things that if everything else was lost and only they remained, it would still mean that your life would be full."

"The pebbles are the other things that matter like your job, your home and your car. The sand is everything else, the small stuff.

If you put the sand into the jar first there is no room for the pebbles or the golf balls." *(There is no room for the physical fitness, health and wellbeing).* The same goes for life. If you spend all your time and energy on the small stuff, you will never have room for the things that are vital to your longevity, health and wellbeing."

The Professors message asks you to pay more attention to the things that are critical to your health and happiness. Take time to be physically active and fit so that you can have the energy to play with your children. To be there for them as they grow up because if you don't take care of your health and fitness, you may not even be fit enough to enjoy life with them later. Take time to keep healthy and get check-ups. Take your partner out to dinner. There will always be time to do the small stuff like clean the house and mow the lawns. Prioritise time for the golf balls first, the things that really matter: your physical health, those that you love and who love you. Set your priorities and "the rest is just sand."

When a student asked what the wine represented. The professor smiled.

"I'm glad you asked. It just goes to show that no matter how full your life may seem, there's always room for a glass of wine with a friend."

◆

I wanted to share an inspiring example of a client of mine who began her unzip the fat suit journey with over 40 kilograms to lose. She had zero desire or motivation to exercise at all. She was extremely unfit, hadn't exercised for about 30 years and could barely walk around her lounge room, let alone do any other form of movement.

At the final stages of writing this book, she is less than 5 kilograms away from her ideal weight, shape and size. Today she is motivated to move her body and follow the commitments. In her words: 'the battle in my head is gone'.

From someone who dreaded going for a walk, she now loves swimming, walking and working out with a personal trainer three to four times per week because she was able to use these strategies to prioritise her 'golf balls'. She made the decision that movement of her body needed to become a 'golf ball' because one of her 'Why's' involved having enough energy to play with and enjoy her grandkids, so she needed to put movement into her 'jar first'.

When I ask her what her opinion about exercise is now she says, "it's one of the most necessary parts of my life, I am now the kind of person who likes to move my body".

The reason I mention this lady here is that one of the key affirmation statements I asked her to begin using early on in her weight reduction journey was: *'I'm the kind of person who enjoys moving my body'*.

When she first began saying this she would nearly choke on the words, she felt resistance and rejection when she said it. She would scoff at the words; she never believed one of them. Now she is genuinely the greatest advocate.

She says, "I kept saying those words and I doubted them. I doubted I could ever believe them let alone do it. Now I AM THAT PERSON! I am the kind of person who loves it. I love exercising, swimming and working out. I love how it makes me feel and I look forward to doing something every day."

To continue reprogramming your mind, begin by repeating this statement regularly throughout the day:

*"I am the kind of person who enjoys moving my body".*

No matter how much resistance there is at first, if you persist in saying it to yourself at least 10 times per day for 30 days, something wonderful will happen. Each time you say it, you will be rewiring your brain for exercise. I've done it, the client I mentioned did it and hundreds of others have done it too. Persist; trust and you will be rewarded with incredible motivation.

I used to hate exercise with a passion, avoid it at all costs and find excuse after excuse. I was the kid I mentioned before. I was the one who came last in athletics on school sport's days. I was chosen last in team sports, and only chosen because the teacher said everyone had to be involved. I would dread PE class. I would cringe in mortification as I waited for someone to choose me to be on his or her team. Not one person chose me unless they had to, sometimes only when urged to by the teacher. For most of the next 25 years of my life, I avoided any form of physical activity at all costs. I believed I was useless and hopeless at it, so I shouldn't even bother trying. My subconscious fear was *'I'll be no good at it anyway, so at least if I don't do it, I won't embarrass myself'*.

Then I learned how to rewire my mind to perceive movement of my body as one of the greatest priorities in my day by doing the exact suggestions I have made to you. I repeated to myself everyday *"I am the kind of person who enjoys moving my body'*. I didn't believe it at first; I scoffed, avoided, procrastinated and used the snooze button till it wouldn't work.

Now I do something that increases my heart rate and strengthens the muscles of my body every day. I was the world's greatest excuse maker; I wasted at least 20 gym memberships over the years and hired umpteen treadmills that were lucky to be used twice.

Now willingly and enjoyably, I workout at least 4 to 5 times per week. On the other days I consciously choose to do at least a half hour of strenuous activity. I wiggle and dance to music for a few minutes every day; I seek out ways to park my car so I can walk further. I choose to make extra trips up and down my stairs at home. I will purposefully do 2 or 3 trips to carry the washing downstairs or to put the ironing away. After going to the supermarket, I will only carry a few shopping bags inside so I can go back to the garage a few times to get the rest.

If the old 'queen of excuses' that was me, can program and rewire this change, anyone can.

Give it a go. Become the kind of person who enjoys moving your body more!

## No More Excuses

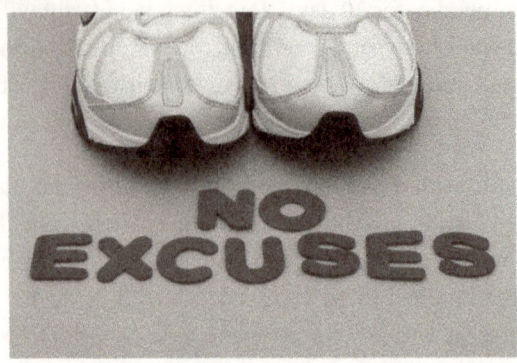

**I'm sure you or someone you know will have used one or two of these excuses in the past.**

What are the excuses you've relied on?

**I don't have the *time***

*This really means I haven't prioritised the time to do this. Other things or people are more important therefore I am not worthy of spending this time on myself. Therefore, I'm not worthy.*

**If your regular excuse is: I don't have the time to exercise or I'm too busy, I suggest you read the metaphor by *Byron Katie: the three types of business and whose business am I In?* (I have provided it in Chapter 11).** I would then ask you to prioritise just 5 - 15 minutes each day at first. I suggest a small amount of time to begin with is better than nothing at all. So make it realistic. When something becomes a priority everyone, can find at least 10 minutes during the day. In that time, commit to doing some form of activity that increases the heart rate. It could be star jumps in the bathroom, if that's all the time you have, or playing three of your favourite tunes and dancing to them.

It can be as simple as setting an alarm on your phone to signal it's time for a few minutes to get down and boogie, to wiggle and move. Commit to do this for a minimum of 7 days. Once you have become used to that 5 - 15 minutes you will naturally find you want to do more. All it takes is starting somewhere.

Then simply assess how you feel, what has changed and what you have achieved in that 7 days. Use that time to check if you have prioritized movement as important enough on your list of life's must do's.

# I can't afford to get healthy

*This really says I think I have to have money to buy the right food or wear the right outfit to the gym in order to get healthy. Instead assess what you can do now, incidental exercise at home, walk around the park or on the beach, swim in the ocean. Find free ways to move the body more, park further from the office and walk the rest of the way. Turn on the radio and dance. Again it is simply about prioritising movement into your day. It doesn't have to cost money, that's an excuse.*

Use what you have around the house, the local park or free exercise videos that can be borrowed from the library or downloaded from www.realage.com

Remember, it doesn't have to cost any money to move your body. You simply need to find free ways to do it. Dance around the house to your favourite music if that rings your bells. Do press ups against your lounge room wall or walk up and down your stairs, if you have them, an extra 10 times each day. It doesn't matter what it is, just *wiggle and move*.

# It's too much effort

*This says I can't be bothered, I'm not motivated, and it's not a priority again. Movement isn't important to me yet.*

Take the time to reconsider your 'Whys'. Go back to the Introduction and Chapter 1. Re-think what is important to you about being slim and healthy. Make it more personal, find a 'Why' that makes your heart sing. Use the suggestions I provided in response to some of the other excuses. Would you rather move your body for 10 minutes a day or be dead for the rest of your life? Can you be bothered now?

# I'll do it later

*And never do! Then probably feel guilty later. Once again, set an alarm on your phone to remind you to allocate time during the day.*

Re-read all the answers I provided as part of the other excuses. This excuse is just a procrastination program hiding the simple fact that, it's not a priority for you yet. Use the Control audio to tap away the 'feeling of resistance or procrastination'. Listen to the *Rewire audios* and the *Motivation to Move my Body and Exercise Program Audio*.

## I'm not sporty or athletic

*This excuse really says I CAN'T therefore I never will. We don't need to be good at sports or athletics to move our body. It can be about fun, not necessarily sports. Why not set a time to research and learn about other fun opportunities to move. It doesn't have to be sport. It could be learning to dance (take a belly or line dancing class or go to the library and take out a training DVD). It could be yoga or Tai Chi. Buddy up with a friend who is at the same skill level and support each other. Download free audios and videos from www.realage.com* and prioritise healthy movement. You might consider researching free walking groups that can help connect you with other people who want to get out and see the world (or at least see your neighbourhood park).

For me taking time to move my body daily has become my 'time out'. I spend an hour or so, 4 to 5 times per week at the gym or walking, without a phone, without emails, without other people needing me. It's my time out; I use that time to listen to the CPR audios, other motivational audios or music. It's a priority for me, and I process how my day will unfold while I'm there.

Barter with a friend who is fit and knows what exercises to do and ask them to teach you. Join walking groups, or laughter clubs or any active group that you resonate with (you'll be surprised who you meet and how much fun it can be).

**What will people think of me? I'm too fat to be seen at the gym or wearing a bathing suit or gym outfits.**

This is usually the fear of making mistakes or fear of what others will think. What if I fail or embarrass myself?

Perhaps it's simply time to focus back on your 'Whys' in order to prioritise your health and decide differently. Remember my client from earlier in the chapter? She used to feel the exact same way and used it as an excuse not to start at all. She eventually started by walking around her lounge room and built up to where she is today.

Quite a few of my clients have used variations of this excuse for a variety of reasons that included:

- "Everyone will be skinny and fit at the gym, I'll stand out"
- "I'm embarrassed about being seen 'wobbling', 'panting' down the street"

- "I don't want to be seen, I feel disgusted that I let myself go"
- "People will stare at my bumps and rolls"

You name it and I have heard it, even worse comments than the ones I have mentioned. The trouble is, when the inner critic goes unchecked with this toxic thinking; it keeps you stuck in the fat suit, locked away feeling worse.

I ask clients to ask themselves these 'ask, answer, discuss' questions:

1. Is this fear moving me towards health?
2. What would my inner coach say/do instead?
3. What would happen if I let that fear go?
4. How would my life and body be different if I did?
5. Am I willing to let it go anyway?
6. What's the worst that could happen if I did go for a walk/to gym?
7. What will happen if I continue to hold onto that fear?
8. Am I going to ever wear my goal outfit and get healthy by not going?
9. What's more important- holding onto the fear or risking the chance that I might actually find health?

Another tip is to use the Control audio for 'feelings'. Repeat it a few times tapping at each point as you say:

- This fear
- This embarrassment
- This worry, what will people think
- This resistance

When you get to the karate chop point remember to say:

*"I let it all go. I don't need it anymore. The past is the past, enough is enough. I give myself permission to be healthy and slim. I can do this, I feel good."*

Ask yourself whether you recognise any of these excuses or, if you have used a particular one often in the past.

What's your excuse …have you been waiting for slim and healthy to come to you?

## Top Tips to Move Your Body More:

- Listen regularly to the Program audio: Motivation to Move your Body & Exercise
- Listen regularly to the Rewire audio: Unzip the fat suit (cardio version)
- Remember to repeat frequently:

*"I'm the kind of person who enjoys moving my body more".*

You don't need to believe it yet, just start saying it and see what happens.

You will be amazed at how easy it becomes, how confident and motivated you will feel.

| Remember your 10 Commitments |
|:---:|
| Rehearse Outfit |
| Audio Daily |
| Weigh Once |
| Stomach chooses |
| Smaller Portions |
| Chew Slowly |
| Push Plate |
| Thirst = Water |
| Wiggle Move |
| Write Progress |

# TEN

## Program Metabolism

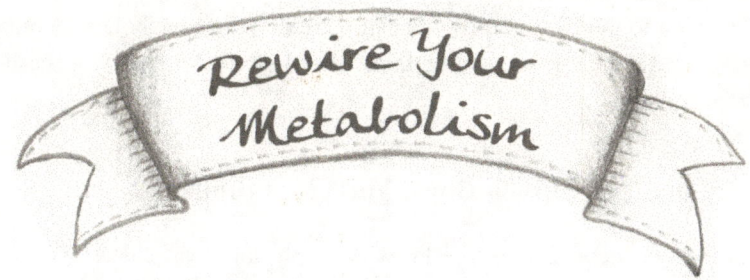

Metabolism: a word that is widely used but do we really know what it is and how to maximise it? Let's see shall we?

Metabolism is a term that refers to the breakdown and transformation of food into energy, so your body can get up and go throughout the day!

Your metabolic rate therefore is the speed at which your body can break down food and absorb nutrients for energy. Your metabolic rate is dependent on many factors including the amount of physical movement you do, your mental and hormonal states (Thyroid function in particular) and many other things.

### Going up:

Your metabolic rate rises at various times. For instance, it increases when you do physical activity, it will also rise if you are anxious.

### Going down:

If your metabolic rate can rise, it can therefore reduce too. Factors that can reduce your metabolic rate are: prolonged starvation, fasting or yo-yo dieting, depression, lethargy, inactivity, hormonal imbalance and a host of other reasons too.

If metabolic rates help you transform food into useful productive energy (burn kilojoules you ingest), then knowing how to increase that rate is important to unzip the fat suit more efficiently. Especially if you are someone who has yo-yo dieted or used starvation 'punishment' diets in the past.

Interestingly, research shows that brainwave states such as meditation (alpha state) and hypnosis (theta state) can increase the metabolic rate too. So using your CPR audios will help to increase your metabolic rate. This is so beneficial that I have included suggestions and techniques within many of the CPR audios to help the subconscious mind boost the immune system and the metabolic rate safely. Just by listening to the CPR audios you can increase your metabolic rate, absorb the nutrients and eliminate the excess faster than before. All the more reason to use the audios daily!

## These are my Top Tips to Boost Your Metabolism

When you follow these tips, excess fat will simply fall away faster, it'll be the easiest thing you'll ever do.

1.  Eat more green leafy vegetables, raw salads and fruit – it takes more energy for the body to digest them, so you'll burn more kilojoules – yippee!
2.  Add chilli and or cayenne pepper to some of your meals. Some of the benefits include increasing your metabolism to assist in weight reduction.
3.  Cumin is said to provide a substantial amount of iron to support energy and metabolism. It also helps digestion by stimulating pancreatic digestive enzymes to help break down food. Hey ho! That's what the metabolism likes to do!
4.  In research studies, green tea extract has been shown to increase metabolism – go figure! Have a cup or 2 a day instead of other caffeine drinks!
5.  Sip warm water with lemon first thing in the morning and throughout the day. This balances alkalinity levels to help keep you healthy
6.  Use the techniques I have mentioned in the book and the CPR audios to take control of unhealthy cravings or head hunger for inappropriate foods. The audios also have specific suggestions to increase metabolism.
7.  Eat smaller portions of food. Sound familiar? Smaller portions are digested more easily; therefore the metabolism can get to work faster.
8.  Chew Slowly! I feel another commitment coming on. When you chew slowly the metabolic rate is easily doing what it does best.

9.   Remember there are no, *'no foods'*, simply less of them and less often.

10.  Choose healthy life giving foods wherever you can. Choose foods grown from the soil, raw foods, natural foods with a variety of colours. Eat a balance of reds, greens and yellows. The more variety of natural colours in the foods you eat the better the balance of nutrients you will be ingesting, the easier the metabolic rate will get to work. Choose a balance of whole grains, proteins, fibres, healthy fats such as avocados, and nuts. General rule: if it's grown from the soil or on plants or trees, it's life-giving food.

11.  Avoid bread and starches. Choose less of them because they are harder to digest, so they slow the metabolic rate.

12.  Avoid sugary processed foods, sweets, pastries and takeaways. Choose less of them and less often (ditto as above).

13.  A large proportion of the population is lactose intolerant. If you are or are concerned that you might be, avoid milk or milk products that contain lactose where you can. If your body finds it hard to process lactose then this will definitely slow the metabolism and therefore, slow your unzip the fat suit progress. Remember, you can get your calcium intake from other sources of natural foods such as almonds, sunflower seeds, brazil nuts and salmon. Also green leafy vegetables including broccoli, kale, spinach, bok choy and other Chinese cabbages.

14.  Avoid alcohol (less of it and less often). Your body has to divert energy from systems such as digestion in order to process and eliminate the toxins in alcohol. If you can't avoid it, then drink a glass of water between each alcoholic beverage. Slow your intake down and give your body the chance to process it. Your metabolic rate, your liver, pancreas and your digestive system will thank you.

15.  Have your main meal of the day in the middle of the day. Food is more easily metabolised when you are active.

16.  Have soup for dinner (with no bread). A lighter meal at the end of the day will be easier for your body to digest and metabolise while you sleep. Sweet dreams!

17.  Include protein with every meal. Choose your protein first then add your vegetables or salad to suit the protein. Proteins can include red and white meats, fish, almonds, seeds and eggs. Remember 'alive foods' from the soil are rich in protein, calcium, fibre and the balance of nutrients we need to be healthy too. Protein helps build muscle mass. They are more easily metabolised and turn into lasting energy. Approximately 50 to 70 grams of protein per meal is adequate.

18. Breakfast is a must to kick start the metabolism first thing! Include a protein; egg on wholegrain toast or muesli with some nuts and seeds or yogurt, nuts and fruit. Yum!

    **Note to self**: when you skip breakfast you'll have a sluggish metabolic rate. Kick the day off with a great start by eating breakfast and burn those kilojoules away easily!

19. Drink at least 2 litres of water each day. You need water for the metabolism to function optimally. Refer back to the commitment about water to remember how important it really is for your brain, bones and body. When you are dehydrated the entire system that is your body finds it harder to do everything it needs to do, including metabolising foods into energy.

20. Drink herbal tea instead of caffeine throughout the day. Peppermint tea will cleanse the palate and is great for digestion.

21. The metabolic rate increases when you move your body more. Hooray! So earn your meals by moving your body first. When you sit down to a meal you'll feel great because you'll know that you've enjoyed moving your body first and it now *needs* nutrition rather than just wants it.

22. Eat regularly. Don't skip meals. Choose 3 small meals each day (refer to Chapter 13, Feed the Body). If your body needs a snack choose a small amount of protein like nuts or seeds.

23. Recognise the difference between greedy appetite and genuine hunger. Commit to do at least three things from the 'Power of Three' list. Determine which type of hunger it is before eating.

24. Ensure your body moves rigorously (raise the heartbeat, raise a sweat) for at least 20 – 40 minutes a day.

25. If you're challenged by 'exercise', then instead say it's 'time to move my body'. Activities like dancing to your favourite tunes, working up a sweat with the vacuum, taking the washing out to the line in 3 or 4 small trips rather than lugging it in one big basket, are all simple examples of how you can move your body more and increase your metabolic rate. Swim, take a Zumba class, do yoga or learn Tai Chi. Use normal activities and put a little more energy into them. Park further away from work and walk the rest of the way. Use the time to 'smell the roses'. Put music on and go wild cleaning the house, de-cluttering the wardrobe or garage. Listen to your favourite tunes and work up a sweat weeding the garden. The more active you are - the faster your metabolism, the faster you absorb nutrients and burn fat.

26. Wash your car with lots of vim and vigour. Soap it up, involve the kids or grandkids, have fun together.
27. Find lots of chores you've been putting off around the home and enjoy feeling the energy you burn.
28. Go for a walk each day, every step you take helps you increase your metabolic rate and walk the kilos away.
29. Listen to the CPR audios. They provide suggestions to help you increase your metabolic rate safely and sensibly too.

**And importantly:**

• 30. Be a better friend to your body and yourself every day. Remind yourself of the good things you've achieved every day. Notice the little successes, the milestones and the natural changes along the way. The more positive you are, the more your body will let excess fat drop away. The calmer you feel, the faster the fat will fall away too. Your state of mind has enormous impact on the state of your health, your digestion and your metabolism. So be happy, kind and compassionate to you!

When you combine some of the ideas above and use the 10 Commitments to find the slim and healthy you, you will be burning, chewing, flushing, eliminating and loving the kilojoules away!

| Remember your 10 Commitments |
|:---:|
| Rehearse Outfit |
| Audio Daily |
| Weigh Once |
| Stomach chooses |
| Smaller Portions |
| Chew Slowly |
| Push Plate |
| Thirst = Water |
| Wiggle Move |
| Write Progress |

# ELEVEN

## Program – Once You Zip it Off - You Can Keep it Off

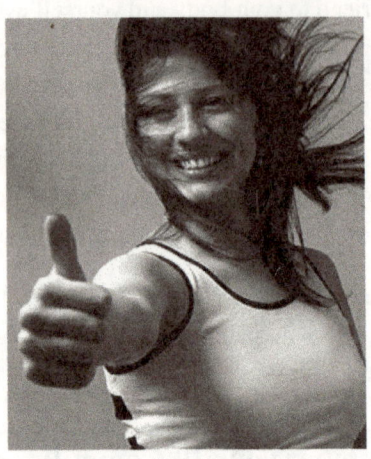

Once you begin to take control of those old eating patterns and move toward your ideal weight, shape and size, it is important to ensure that you have a belief, a 'knowing' deep inside, that the slim and healthy you is permanent.

Many people have become so used to unhelpful self-talk - inner critic programs, that self-doubt niggles away at the back of their mind, even when they're doing well. *"What if the weight comes back?"* or *"But I lost weight before and I put it back on"* or *"I'll never keep this off"*.

If this is the case, it's time to feel great because this unhelpful self-talk can be successfully dealt with using the techniques discussed in the book so far and one or two other 'magic' keys I still have for you.

Remember, all thoughts (even the self-doubt ones) are simply neural pathways in the brain that can be interrupted, re-programmed and rewired. Just because you have a thought, doesn't mean its real, true or permanent. You now have the strategies to interrupt thoughts and switch on better ones. It doesn't even matter if your mind doesn't believe the new ones yet, just keep thinking confident thoughts, and your brain learns through repetition to believe them. You can do that! Yeah!

## The keys to being slim and healthy permanently:

1. Be alert for the inner critic. Be mindful of unhelpful self-talk (doubt, fear, 'what if's') and use your *Inner Coach* to reframe what the slim and healthy you would say. Do this every day. Keep mind rehearsing far into your future with images of the slim and healthy you. See yourself slim and making great decisions about food and your body in 5 years, 10 years. Imagine it as far into the future as you can. See it, feel it and pretend it as if it is already real. Pretend interactions with loved ones as a slim and healthy person. Remember, you are programming your mind for permanent change. You do this through repetition and heightened feel good sensations, because they help your brain learn!

2. Use your CPR Mind Potential Kit audios as often as you need and for as long as you like. When you continue to use these audios (and others from the website www.thepotentialist.com if you wish) then you will continue to control, program and rewire your mind and habits to create the slim and healthy you permanently. Remember there are so many other benefits to the CPR audios including lowering blood pressure, reducing unhealthy cholesterol levels, developing a more positive outlook, sleeping better and creating a more balanced sense of wellbeing.

3. Continue to follow the 10 Commitments every day. If you ever find yourself slipping or doubting again, I can guarantee you won't have been doing ALL the Commitments. Check them and be honest with yourself. Sometimes you think you are doing them and actually you've let one or two slip. Recommit by signing the Commitment statements again. Always come back to the 10 Commitments. Use your CPR Audios. Re-read the book and all the exercises again; people get different messages from the book every time they read it. You'll succeed every time you refocus.

4. In order to be healthy, always consult your stomach for what it needs to eat and the quantity. Trust your stomach, it will always indicate what it needs when you consult it about food choices and quantities. It will feel light when the choice is nutrition and heavy or uncomfortable if it is a greedy appetite or head hunger choice. From today, commit to never consulting your head, mouth or eyes about what you eat again. Your body wants, needs and responds positively to nutritious foods. Your head,

eyes and mouth are susceptible to the lies you told yourself in the past. Your head, mouth and eyes are where inner conflict, the old potential head battles about food existed. The battle was never in the stomach it was always above the neck. Unfortunately it was below the neck where the consequences of your heads' choices were stored. (As fat around the hips, on the tummy, bum, legs and arms). So the only way to be sure you are behaving as a slim and healthy person is to always ask, listen to and believe your stomach when it comes to food. When you make this permanent shift, you become the kind of person who is slim and healthy always.

5.  Use the *'I'm gorgeous: You're Gorgeous'* confidence building techniques from Chapter 7. When doing your mirror work, you can exchange 'I'm gorgeous/ you're gorgeous' for: *'I believe in me/I believe in you'.* You can also exchange what you say in the mirror with *'I'm the kind of person who is slim and healthy'.*

    Remember just like the: **'I'm the kind of person who enjoys moving my body'** rewire statement, when you say it often enough, you create a new electrical circuitry, the wiring in your brain. This is essentially a new memory. Reinforce it often enough and it becomes a belief, an inner knowing.

6.  Listen to the Build Confidence Rewire audios regularly. They continue to reinforce how amazing you really are. The more you hear that, the more you learn to know it and feel it too.

7.  Remember to increase your adversity quotient by finding ways to become like the coffee bean. Look for how to enhance circumstances, people and events rather than blame, react or sabotage. Develop resilience by always looking for the wisdom instead of only focusing on the 'hurt'. Take responsibility for your own part in a drama, habit or attitude.

    Ask yourself *"What can I learn from this event, circumstance or person?"* or *"How can I respond differently this time?"* Use the 'Power of Three List' to interrupt the inner critic crap and repeat: "I can do this" x 10.

8.  Stay in your own business. I'll explain this concept in a moment. Suffice it to say for now, when you distract yourself and 'busily' get into someone else's business, you can end up using other people's 'needs or emotional stuff' as an excuse to stop prioritising your health. You end up putting your needs on the back burner again.

When you **stop** using other people's business as an excuse for not having time to do yours, you finally break old sabotage patterns. You can have healthy compassion for others, but also the time to take action for yourself too.

## The Magic Key of all Keys:

**Use the special 'You Can Do It' Control audios**

**Control & Conquer Self Doubt & the Fear of Yo-Yo Dieting**

**Control & Conquer Self Blame - I Believe in Me/Once it's Off I Keep it Off**

1. Use these Control audios as often as you need to eliminate doubts for good. Build self-belief that the slim and healthy you is here permanently. These audios also deal with forgiving yourself for gaining weight or if you've ever yo-yo dieted.
2. Use the *Build Confidence Rewire audios* too. They will help you become the kind of person who believes in 'you'. You will be a person who has compassion, respect and honours your own needs too. You can become the kind of person who chooses to be slim and healthy, who treats your body with love and respect, not because you have to, but because you deserve it and want it too.

If you need help with this drop me an email: info@thepotentialist.com

## Staying in Your Own Business

A few years ago I read a story by the wonderful author and personal development guru, Byron Katie. To this day her story is still, for me, one of the best ways to explain the importance of prioritising time for you, your health and body.

Once you do prioritise your health needs you find that you also have so much more energy and time to give other people too. You also develop a deeper understanding of what you can change, what you can't, and what you can accept the way that it is. This helps eliminate feelings of resentment and unhelpful emotions that can keep you zipped in the fat suit, playing out old sabotage eating patterns.

It is my hope that understanding this helps you understand that your role is not always to provide solutions for everybody's problems, it is to be compassionate, guiding and supportive, while others learn how to help themselves.

Byron Katie's story helped me identify the tasks and people that I had inadvertently used as an excuse to hold me back from achieving the healthier me. I would keep myself busy taking on other people's responsibilities, I would avoid the responsibility I had to my own health.

If we have a tendency to do this, we can unconsciously stop another person from growing and learning their life lessons. In our misguided desire to 'protect' others and be the 'saviour', we can stop him or her from learning what he or she needed to learn in order to be the best version of themselves that they could be too.

**We therefore stop ourselves from being the best version of our self too.**

Byron Katie suggests that there are three kinds of business *"mine, yours, and God's."* She says that, *"God's business is anything that's out of our control such as the weather, earthquakes or when you or I will die."*

She believes *(and I concur)* that most of our unhelpful emotional stress comes from *"living in someone else's business"*. Her concept suggests therefore, that if we are busy being in someone else's business, we are not living in and working through our own.

Every time we experience an unhelpful emotional state, Byron Katie suggests, we are not in our own business; we are in someone else's.

Remember one of my 'alarm' phrases in Chapter 5? *"I should"*? Alarm phrases like the ones I mentioned in that chapter can also alert you to the fact that you are about to get into someone else's business, and when you do, it leaves you feeling an unhelpful emotional reaction.

The difference here, is that the alarm phrases to look out for are things like: *"he should"*, *"she should"*, or *"I wish he or she would"* or *"You don't do or say this...", "why can't you do or say that...", "you need to...' or "why don't you..."* the list could go on.

Every time you wish that something or someone else were different, even if you believe it is for their own good, you are in their business. You are not only keeping yourself from your own business, you are also stopping them from learning how to grow, by dealing with their own business.

Byron Katie suggests that every time she has been in someone else's business she experienced an unhelpful emotional state of loneliness, separation or hurt. She said *"If you are living your life and I am mentally living your life, who is here living mine?... I am separate from myself, wondering why my life doesn't work."*

In my experience I agree with her theory. Whenever I think about the loneliest or most emotionally 'toxic' times of my life, I can link those times to 'wishing and wanting someone else or life to be 'better', 'different' 'happier', more this or more that.

Byron suggests, *"The next time you're feeling stress or discomfort, ask yourself whose business you're in mentally, and you may burst out laughing!"*

If you do find yourself in an unhelpful emotional state, this is a wonderful question to ask of yourself, *"Whose business am I in?"*

I have told Byron Katie's story to many clients who are on the *'unzip the fat suit'* journey. I use it especially with people who have 'busy' lives and find no time to prioritise their own health or movement of their body. They make all kinds of verbal commitments to take action, but week after week the excuses pile up. *"My daughter needed this..." "My husband wanted that... my church group this..."* or *"I didn't get a chance to walk because my friend needed that..."*

When we are in other people's business we disempower them, we stop them from experiencing the lessons they need to learn in order to become a better person. Doing this can potentially cause two important issues:

1.  You feel stuck in a rut or eventually resentful that you have no time for yourself

2.  They feel stifled and don't grow or can build an expectation that 'you'll always do it anyway'. This means they never learn how to build resilience for life either. Their AQ never increases, because you always fix it for them.

When you choose to always be responsible for other people's business, all your time is taken up with that and you de-prioritise your own growth and health too.

An example of this occurred a few years ago with a client who repeatedly lost a few kilos and then put them back on. For a year she hovered around the same weight within 5 or 6 kilos. It wasn't until I read her this story by Byron Katie that she realised what she had been doing.

Her husband was addicted to alcohol. He was making promises to deal with the addiction but week after week, nothing changed. If he'd binged the night before she would give up her days to drive him to work. She would fear he would lose his licence and therefore their business would suffer if he were still over the legal alcohol limit. So with good intent, she would try to protect him by spending her days taking him from job to job.

She kept giving up her plan to exercise or go for a walk, so she could spend the whole day driving him around.

By the time I saw her again she had regained the weight and had become depressed, angry and a little resentful. Her husband was still addicted to alcohol, because there were no consequences for him, no reason to stop. She made it all okay for him to keep drinking. I was also seeing the husband for alcohol addiction and he said to me during a session one day: *'My wife will drive me around tomorrow so there's no reason why I can't have a drink tonight'.*

I convinced him to repeat what he had told me to his wife. When she heard this she broke down in tears and finally saw what she had been doing. By continually trying to 'protect' him, she realised she had actually disempowered him and assisted his addiction.

That very day she apologised for being in his business and vowed she would support him as much as she could, but she could not drive him around again. He now knew if he wanted to keep his licence and the business, he had to take responsibility.

After a couple of weeks he made further appointments to see me and eventually took control of his life. He thanked me for reading the story to his wife because it inspired her to care for herself, and forced him to face his own consequences. His wife succeeded in her goal for her healthy weight, shape and size.

- She learned to take responsibility for her own motivation, exercise and health. She stopped using his addiction as an excuse to ignore her own health needs.
- Her husband took responsibility for his own business and his sobriety.
- Their relationship flourished. There was now mutual respect for each other's individual needs and life lessons.

If you find you never have time for you, or you realise you are using other people as an excuse not to do what you need to do for your health, then perhaps it's simply time to ask yourself:

- Whose business am I in?
- Am I potentially disempowering anyone?
- How can I guide and support without disempowering either of us?

| Remember your 10 Commitments |
|---|
| Rehearse Outfit |
| Audio Daily |
| Weigh Once |
| Stomach chooses |
| Smaller Portions |
| Chew Slowly |
| Push Plate |
| Thirst = Water |
| Wiggle Move |
| Write Progress |

# TWELVE

## Feed the Soul - Unzip Stress and Rewire Calm

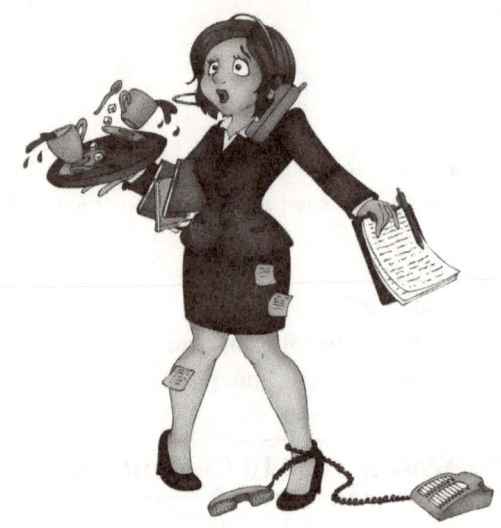

In Chapter 8, I mentioned the importance of de-stressing in relation to our digestive system, and I suggested specific chewing techniques to support this process. However, making a commitment to manage stress on a daily basis is vitally important for other reasons too.

Remember if you are stressed when you eat or if you eat fast or on the run, you create a stressful internal environment and your digestive system switches off in order to manage the fight, flight or freeze (FFF) response.

Your body doesn't reactivate digestion properly until you have calmed down and switched off the 'danger' mode. The benefits of stress management are obvious to most of us without saying anything more, however I am going to expand this issue a little further for a number of reasons. It is not simply your digestive system that is affected by stress; your immune system, hormonal system and memory are adversely affected as well.

Stress affects your overall brain function and critical thinking processes, the health of your skin, growth of your hair and the longevity and health of your organs. Even the health of your relationships can suffer when stress levels are high.

It is reported in some medical fields that 75 to 85% of illness or the symptoms of illness are either caused or exacerbated by stress. Some in the medical arena have even suggested that figure might be as high as 90%.

From personal experience, and having witnessed the experiences of many of my clients, I agree with the 90% ratio. Having dealt with autoimmune issues for over 25 years now, I am aware of how imperative it is to reduce internal and external stress in order that the symptoms of the disease are reduced too. During stressful times in my life, the symptoms have flared. When my life, my mind, body and spirit were in harmony, the symptoms reduced and eventually disappeared, the medical markers normalised.

**Importantly:**

**The ease and speed with which you unzip the fat suit is severely affected by stress**

Aside from general health issues, stressed people find it more challenging to unzip the fat suit too. The calmer you remain, the easier and faster weight reduction will be. The calmer you remain, the more enjoyable the journey to slim and healthy will be too.

Even science supports the use of techniques such as self-hypnosis programs to reduce stress and reduce weight more effectively. CPR Mind Potential Audios take you to the self-hypnosis brainwave state. A weight reduction trial carried out by Friedman and Taub compared self-hypnosis techniques with other stress reduction techniques, including biofeedback. Those participating in the trial were either given self-hypnosis or biofeedback techniques to use during their weight loss program. Some people were asked to use both techniques. All groups had a significant reduction in blood pressure. However, at six-month follow-up, only patients receiving hypnosis techniques had maintained the reduction in weight. (1) (2)

References: (1) Friedman, H. &Taub, H. (1977). "The Use of Hypnosis and Biofeedback Procedures for Essential Hypertension." International Journal of Clinical and Experimental Hypnosis, 25, 335-347. (2) Friedman, H. &Taub, H. (1978). "A Six Month Follow-up of the Use of Hypnosis and Biofeedback Procedures in Essential Hypertension." American Journal of Clinical Hypnosis, 20, 184-188

# The Importance of Managing Stress

## Remember from Chapter 8?

When you experience stress, w*eight gain* is exacerbated because your sympathetic nervous system (FFF) is dominant in the stress state. A dominance of cortisol (Neurochemical released in FFF) in high stress periods, causes weight gain….d'oh!

- So you can stress yourself *into* keeping the fat suit on or
- You can relax yourself out of it. Yeehah!

If the CPR audios take you automatically into a brainwave state such as self hypnosis, and these states have been proven to reduce stress levels, then using these audios on your journey to unzip the fat suit is a key to allowing the excess kilos to drop away easily.

Stress management is so important to your unzip the fat suit journey, that I have provided a 'Be Stress Free' Program audio. *(If you haven't already started to use it, then start today).*

The calmer you are, the easier becoming slimmer and healthier will be. We know from earlier in the book that our *CPR Mind Potential Audios* allow your brainwaves to slow to the Alpha and Theta states. We also know from our brainwave chart that in those states we enter an internally focused calm state that hovers between meditation and hypnosis. So each time we use the CPR audios we are entering brainwave states that have been proven to reduce stress, and therefore reduce cortisol levels. This of course, leads to the ability to reduce weight more easily.

So now that we know how important reducing stress is to your unzip the fat suit journey, I have provided a number of stress reduction tips for you to choose from (including of course our Be Stress Free Program audio).

# Top Tips to Manage Stress

1.  Imagine a peaceful place, a happy and peaceful space; pretend it is real in your mind. Feel it, see it with all of your senses. Remember your mind doesn't know the difference between real and imagined. You can pretend to be in a relaxed space even if the world around you is chaotic. When you do this, your *'Pharmacist'* will release the right Neuro-chemicals to help calm the body.

2.  5-0 Relax Technique used by an American therapist called Devin Hastings. Devin's technique involves counting backwards from 5 down to zero. Start by saying 5 quite loudly and with as much enthusiasm as if you are stressed. Then as you reduce the numbers, you reduce the intensity of the tone of voice and the volume too. By the time you are down to 3 or 2 you are speaking quietly. When you get to zero you almost whisper it. The more calmly you speak, the more the stress dissolves out of the body. Your whole body will feel as though it is relaxing and dropping in intensity. Once you get to zero, say 'I have permission to relax' x 3 times.

3.  Use the Stress Buster cheat sheet tapping points as you repeatedly say: 'I feel calm, I am calm' at each point.

4.  Imagine or pretend that you are doing the tapping exercise (the mind won't know the difference). This will help to rebalance your nervous system, allowing you to feel calmer.

5.  Take 3 - 6 deep belly breaths every hour.

6.  Visualise turning the stress levels down in the control room of your mind. I refer to the control room in Program audio one: Eliminate Greedy Appetite.

7.  Focus on your breathing then imagine or remember a perfect day, in a perfect place in nature.

8.  Imagine writing the word 'RELAX' or 'CALM' in the air in front of you.

9.  Walk for pleasure. Take your shoes off and feel the grass/sand between your toes.

10. Use the Be Stress Free Program Audio. Use any other Program audio.

11. Laugh more or join a laughter club. According to Dr Caroline Leaf in her book: *Who Switched off My Brain*, laughter reduces stress hormones and relaxes you. A good belly laugh can make the stress hormone cortisol drop by 39% and adrenaline drop by 70%. Laughter also increases the feel good hormone endorphin by 29%. Growth hormones also skyrocket by 87%. Laughter also boosts your immune system. Now that'll inspire you to laugh and keep you healthy and relaxed.

12. De-clutter your house, office, desk, wardrobe, and bookshelf. When you are surrounded by physical clutter, you will subconsciously create a more stressful environment on the inside too. So de-stress your outside world, and you will instantly de-stress your inner clutter too.

13. Imagine breathing in a peaceful colour.

14. Close your eyes and scan your body with your internal mind's eye. Find the calmest place within or on your body. There will be one I promise.

Focus on that calm place and when you feel ready, expand it slowly to cover the whole body with calmness.

15. Be in nature as often as you can.

16. Take a walk at lunchtime. Leave the office, stretch and move your body more throughout the day.

17. Speak to yourself in a calm inner voice that is gentle and kind. Tell yourself regularly throughout the day in this calm and kind voice "I have permission to be calm" or "I feel good".

18. Acknowledge what is genuinely your stress and manage it with the above tips. Acknowledge what is other people's stress (or business), and calmly hand it back to them in your mind.

19. Prioritise at least 10-15 minutes to yourself every day. Whether it is to sit on a park bench and breath deeply or swing on a swing, make it your 'me' time. Even if you have to stop the car on the way home from work for 15 minutes and contemplate or meditate. Just de-clutter your thoughts and breathe deeply as you switch off from the day.

20. Listen to a Program audio every day. Your central nervous system will thank you because listening to the audio puts you into the rest and di-gest (R/D) state. Remember this state allows the body and mind to calm and the digestive system to function properly. This will help you release excess fat easily, reduce cortisol and adrenalin levels and relax more.

21. Ask for help around the home and the office.

22. Nurture yourself for at least an hour a week by yourself for yourself. Have a massage, swim, pamper, counselling, time out to read a good book, meditate, do art, listen to your favourite music or watch a feel good movie.

23. Do a friend audit annually (work out if anyone leaves you feeling drained or bad about yourself). Ask yourself if you are in their busi-ness? If so, are you willing to step out of their business and let them grow? Ask them to support you more or request that they stop saying unhelpful things to you. Ask yourself the 'ask, answer, discuss' ques-tions from Chapter 5. Questions like: am I willing to stop allowing their unhelpful comments or behaviour to influence me? Am I willing to say no appropriately to them or limit the amount of time I spend with them if they persist doing or saying unhelpful things? What would hap-pen if I let this person or their unhelpful limiting beliefs, behaviour or comments go? Am I able to stop letting their unhelpful limiting beliefs, behaviours or comments influence me? What can I do to feel more in control of our encounters?

24. Last thing before bedtime, imagine pressing the release mechanism in the control room of your mind, release all the tension of the day from your body, sense, feel or imagine it draining away.

25. Don't wait to be told! Make these things a priority before somebody else recognises the stress and burnout in you.

26. Seek help: If it is all too much and you don't know where to start, you're already in burnout, get the help you need.

27. Rather than simply accept stressful thoughts and actions, challenge them by asking:

   - What is really going on here?
   - What can I do to feel more in control in this situation?
   - What would my inner coach do or say instead?
   - Whose business am I in?
   - Is the issue/feeling solvable now?
     - If it is solvable, do so by using the CPR audios or another technique from the book.
     - If the issue or feeling is not solvable right now, you can choose to let go of the stressful worry about it by accepting what you can't change just yet and changing what you can. Use a control audio to tap away the stress. Use any of the other stress reduction techniques in this list.

28. Remember you have tools to change your reaction. You can't change others but you can change your response to them.

29. When your "plate" is already full and before your stress metre starts blowing steam, don't be afraid to say no to people (pleasantly of course). You can't help anyone, including yourself, if you burn out or get stress-sickness.

30. Learn to meditate. Starting with 10 minutes a day is all it takes just by focusing on your in breath and out breath. Allow thoughts to flow without focusing on them. Just notice thoughts without judging them. They are simply electrical circuitry in the brain. Notice that and come back to focusing on your breath.

31. Close your eyes and listen to your favourite music that brings joy to your soul.

32. Close your eyes and remember the most peaceful or relaxing day of your life

**Remember:**

*If you haven't already done so, start using your Be Stress Free Program audio, because a calm you is a happier, slimmer and healthier you!*

| Remember your 10 Commitments |
|:---:|
| Rehearse Outfit |
| Audio Daily |
| Weigh Once |
| Stomach chooses |
| Smaller Portions |
| Chew Slowly |
| Push Plate |
| Thirst = Water |
| Wiggle Move |
| Write Progress |

# THIRTEEN

## Feed the Body

### 12 Steps to Healthy Eating and Perfect Athleticism

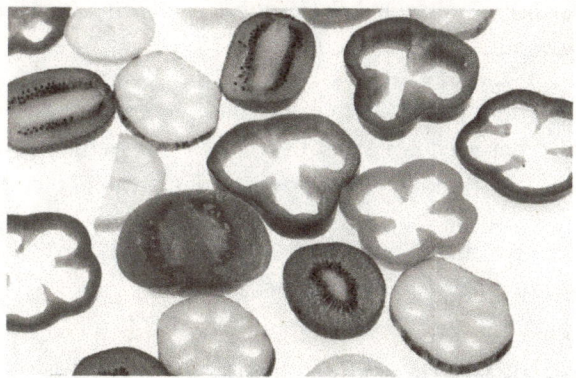

You may have gathered by now, that I take an approach to changing eating patterns and unzipping the fat suit for good that considers all perspectives: mind, body and soul. When these three operate in harmony, the battle in your head is over and you create permanent change.

Throughout the book, I have repeatedly addressed how to work on the unhelpful issues that originate in the mind. I've addressed certain aspects of nutrition in Chapter 10 with the intent of using certain foods or spices to increase the metabolic rate; I've even addressed the 'soul' part of you, the essence that is you by dealing with managing stress factors and building innate confidence. Now it is also vitally important to address how you *feed your physical body* with regard to the overall process of unzipping the fat suit for good.

This chapter encompasses all aspects of feeding the body in nutrition, thought and action. I consider the importance of how we think about what our body is, what it looks like and of course, what we put into it, as imperative to the whole slim and healthy picture.

As mentioned in Chapter 8, renegade fitness experts: Sharny and Julius Kieser have generously provided their unique approach to nutrition, fitness and weight reduction. Their approach is taking the world by storm and I am grateful to them for offering their expertise in this chapter.

The key to their work is very simple. They not only have a gift for helping people obtain peak fitness, they have a gift for making previously challenging information, simple and most importantly: doable. They are straight talking people. They say it like it is which can sometimes be confronting, but what they say is honest and helpful.

They are best selling authors and their current books include: *Never Diet Again – Escape the Diet Trap Forever* and *FITlosophy 1 – Chasing Physical Perfection in a World of Gluttony*.

Neither Sharny nor Julius is afraid to say it like it is. Often they create controversy by saying it that way. For a full list of their best selling books and programs please refer to their biographies provided at the end of the book or go to: www.sharnyandjulius.com.

For now let's focus on their 12-Step Program

## 12 Steps to Healthy Eating and Perfect Athleticism
### *By Renegade Fitness Experts: Sharny and Julius Kieser*

You are an athlete. You're not a fatty. You never were. Even at your darkest day, stomach stretched tight with that familiar discomfort of food pain, the slow death of overeating not only consuming your health, but poisoning your mind. Even then, you were an athlete; you simply didn't know it yet.

Are we wrong? Surely we're predisposed to obesity. It must be genetic. We're fat because of fast food companies, it's a faulty metabolism, its supermarkets, it's mum's fault, tempting television commercials made it happen, that's it. I bet they all have something to do with this mine truck tyre you're carrying around your waist and your bum!

Sharny and I used to think like this, we used to blame everyone and everything around us for the fact that we were in the fat suit. It worked too, for a few years, that was, until we decided we shouldn't kid ourselves anymore and we should eliminate false excuses.

## Excuse one: Fast Food

"Today is going to be the day that we'll finally stumble upon that mad scientist out the back of the fast food outlet *force feeding* children with fatty, greasy, sugary crap that makes them fat." Twenty minutes later, having found no such beast, we would roll out of the fast food joint, straw angrily probing through the ice in our cups, bellies full of 'research', chins greasy. "Nope, they didn't force feed us... they can't be to blame".

It took us a while before we fessed up; we were unfortunately too clever to blame them. We may have been gluttons, but we weren't stupid. Not one fast food joint force-fed us the crap. They didn't send fatty feeding parties into our homes and cram the junk down our children's throats; they didn't drag us in off the street and tie us to the seat drip-feeding us till we tipped the scales at our peak. We walked in, we paid cash, we chewed, we swallowed, and we smiled and did it again. Damn it. The logic was too sound.

*We chose t*o eat the junk; they weren't giving it away free, we actually paid for it. Hell, we even paid for the upsize just to be sure. And then we got the second dinner box for the "visiting relatives" and the 'happy' fatty meal for our kids. Might as well fatten them up too!

## Excuse two: It's Genetic

Julius' brothers are skinny, so the reason for the fat can't be genetics. Hang on, hang on. I know. I bloody well know who is to blame for this fat!! It's my mum!

## Excuse three: It's my *mother's* fault...

Oh no ... we're too clever for this one too. Let's address this excuse by looking at our 12 steps to healthy eating and perfect athleticism

## Step 1: Blame your mother...

We're joking. You can't blame her for this. Remember she's the one who nagged you to eat your veggies?

## The Real Step 1: Take Responsibility

It's your fault you're fat. We're not even going to sugar-coat it. You'll probably eat it.

Just teasing. Remember, we've been there too and so has Maggie Wilde. This is simply about deciding to stop blaming anyone or anything and choosing to accept responsibility for what you can change, what goes into your mouth and how you move your body. If you're challenged in this area, use the CPR – Mind Potential audios Maggie provides to help overcome the subconscious blocks. They can help control and eliminate any cravings till you're back in control of your choices.

So here goes:

**Here's the remainder of our 12 steps to healthy eating and perfect athleticism:**

## Step 2: Change your perspective – never say that you are fat again

*A rock, lying immobile on a riverbed for years and years gets covered in a thick layer of moss. Is it a rock, or is it now moss?*

It *looks* like a ball of moss, but it's not moss. It's a rock. If the rock had eyes and could look in the mirror, it would only see moss. But luckily for the rock, there are no mirrors and it has no eyes. To the rock, it is still a rock, covered in moss. To the outside world (you and me) we know it is still a rock, just covered in moss. In fact it can never ever be *called* moss. It can never *be* moss.

So if the rock were to say "I'm moss," we would all just think him a fool, correct?

Saying "I'm fat" is no different. You're not fat. You can't be. The fat that has collected on your body is a result of lying immobile on your metaphoric riverbed for years. You are the rock, and the fat is your moss.

You cannot ever call yourself fat. According to this theory, if you call yourself fat, then I'll call you a fool.

Remember Maggie Wilde has said throughout this book that our brains do not know the difference between real and imagined, so if you continue to call yourself fat… then your mind will help you achieve it! Your brain will continue to believe it, your metabolic rate will continue in its lethargy, your motivation will stay low and you'll continue to stay in the fat suit.

208

So what do you call yourself?

Imagine if you could get instant, painless liposuction to rid your body of all of the fat, you would look like bones, muscle, organs, and skin - no fat.

*You'd look like an Olympic athlete.*

And that is what you should call yourself. Say it now.

*"I'm not fat, I'm an athlete, covered in a layer of fat."*

Call it a winter coat. All you have to do now is lose the winter coat.

And do you know what? Being heavy has given you the best foundation for athleticism you could ever hope for.

When we train professional athletes, one of the most effective things we do to improve their strength and endurance is to have them train in a weighted vest. Anywhere from 10kg to 20kg strapped to their torso is highly effective at turbo charging their fitness. The heart and lungs become devastatingly effective. The joints become more powerful and injury resistant and the muscles efficient and the blood flow strong.

You have been living your life with a weight vest on. It's simply time to take it off or, as Maggie Wilde would say: unzip it!

Believe me when I say this, some of the best athletes we've ever trained have been obese immediately preceding the decision to become athletic. Strip the fat off them, and you have yourself *a powerful warhorse with a heart that can carry it across continents.*

## Step 3: Realise you are an athlete - a damn powerful one!

So... You're not fat; you're an athlete with a winter coat of fat. How do you lose the fat then? Diet or exercise?

Exercise does not burn fat. Exercise does this:

1. Exercise increases your metabolic rate (releases feel good chemicals in the brain and increases the speed at which you metabolise food)
2. Exercise helps you feel good about yourself (positive endorphins in the brain flow more readily after exercise)

3. Exercise prevents your body from burning / eating muscle (you get fitter and build stamina)
4. Exercise releases other Neuro-chemicals that help stimulate learning and memory (remember Maggie's Chapter 9)

Every day, just to survive, your body needs fuel to live. Breathing, walking, thinking; these are all things that require energy that your body has to find from somewhere. Until now, you've got this energy from the food you have eaten. If you eat less, your body gets this energy from your body. It burns or metabolises (eats) fat and muscle.

## *So Exercising a Muscle Essentially takes it Off the Menu*

We don't want to lose the muscle, because muscle needs energy to survive. The less muscle you have, the less energy you need to survive. When we exercise and use our muscles, all that's left for your body to burn/metabolise is the food and nutrients you eat. If you are eating a reduced food intake, then the body will make up the shortfall and burn/metabolise your body's excess fat stores (the winter coat starts to shrink).

Use all the muscles in your body daily to take them off the menu and put excess fat on the menu. Running, swimming, climbing, playing with kids are all fantastic ways to use all the muscles in your body. You don't even have to do much, you just have to do enough exercise to send the message to the body: *I need this muscle, don't eat it.*

## Step 4: Exercise *all the muscles* in your body to prevent them being 'eaten'.

You don't need to exercise for hours at a time. What if you could get the same result in less time?

Well, you can.

The focus is to workout ALL the muscles in your body. Whether it takes you 3 minutes or 60 minutes, make those minutes meaningful. Remember take responsibility for those minutes and work *all* the muscles hard to take them off the menu. When you eat less (smaller portions) and you move your muscles more, you reduce weight because the excess fat is on the menu not your muscle!

## Step 5: Only exercise for as long as you need - only do more if you're enjoying it.

Only do more if you enjoy it. If enjoying exercise challenges you, use Maggie Wilde's Program audio 'Motivation to Exercise & Move Your Body' to change your perspective and enjoy it more. Use her *Rewire* audios too for the best outcome.

## Step 6: Prevent yourself from ever gaining weight again, *then* work on losing what you've stored.

Now, before you even think about *losing* weight, you have to think about how to *prevent yourself from ever gaining any more weight*. Sounds simple right? Sounds logical?

How do you do that? Start by quitting sugar. Sugar, of any kind, is the devil.

We have been led to believe that fat makes you fat. It's the premise behind the "low fat" revolution.

Eating excess fat makes you store it, definitely. But have you tried to eat plain fat. How much butter can you eat with a spoon? Probably just one spoon before you feel too sick.

Now add sugar. Cake icing is just butter and sugar. Add sugar to butter and you can eat a whole tub of it. Fat does make you fat, but sugar is *the delivery mechanism*. Sugar is the taste stimulator. *Sugar makes it easier to eat more of everything*. Why do you think fast food places serve sodas with every meal and add sugar to their burger buns?

Cut out all forms of sugar from your diet and you simply won't eat as much, you won't be able to.

And yes, there is a lot of sugar in fruit. If you really want to lose weight, you'll cut out fruit. But what about the antioxidants? Vegetables are a far more stable, higher source of antioxidant food than fruit.

## Step 7: Quit Sugar – it's the delivery mechanism that makes you eat more and get fat

Sugar is more addictive than heroin.

It's not easy to quit sugar. But it's not easy for anybody to quit sugar, you're not the only one addicted, and you're not the only one who has had to quit. If you're challenged here use Maggie's control cravings audios, you'll be back in control in no time.

Every time you feel like you have to have some sugar, remind yourself that millions of far weaker, less intelligent, less able people have managed to quit. And it's not a life long fight. It only takes a few minutes, sometimes-even seconds if you use the CPR Mind Potential control craving audios.

## Step 8: Cheating is for losers. You're a winner.

What about cheat days?

Sugar is an addictive substance that you have been abusing. Think about yourself as a rehab patient. Do heroin addicts get a cheat day?

## Step 9: Don't fatten up your meals with starch

We're sorry to tell you this, but second to sugar comes starchy carbs. Potatoes, pastas, rices, breads. If you can think of starchy carbs as millions of pieces of sugar stuck together, you'd be close enough to the truth.

Rice, pasta, potatoes and bread provided calories to foot soldiers to allow them to march 40-50 km per day in full armour. The closest we get to that is marching from the supermarket to the car, and we get frustrated if it's further than about 40 metres. God forbid we have to carry our groceries - that's too much to ask!

Cut out the starchy carbs, you're not a foot soldier from the 1900's. The bonus is that your shopping bags will be lighter.

## Step 10: Additives are unpredictable

Additives, colours, preservatives, flavour enhancers. These **are not foods**, they are chemicals disguised as numbers and fancy names that you've been misled to accept that they belong in foods. They're not made in the kitchen or grown in the soil or found on trees. They're concocted in a laboratory. They're chemicals.

Eating unknown chemicals will give you unexpected results. Mix them together and you could have a belly swell and headache of atomic proportions.

## Step 11: Google MSG

The subject of MSG could fill an encyclopaedia, so we recommend Googling MSG and doing your own research. In short, MSG is a flavour enhancer. It brings out the flavour in all foods, so it is in a lot of foods. *MSG also happens to be used to fatten lab rats for obesity research.*

You see, rats aren't normally fat. You have to fatten them up if you want to do obesity research on them. How do you make a rat obese very quickly? Feed it MSG of course (then don't tell anyone who might be eating it).

So get to know the numbers and the acronyms that are used to 'hide' MSG. 621, mono sodium glutamate... Google them all.

## Step 12: Food is fuel, not entertainment.

Oh... my... goodness. What can I eat; you've basically told me I can't eat anything!!

When an alcoholic quits drinking, do they ask "what *can* I drink?" No, they assess "what drink would a sober person drink?"

The way your food has treated your body until now is clearly not serving you. The types of foods you've been eating are making you fatter and fatter, all while robbing you of energy. You need a full review of your consumption.

**Ask yourself:** *"What food would a healthy athlete eat?"*

Vegetables, meat, eggs, nuts and seeds. You are an athlete now, so eat like one. Do this and your body will pay you back with interest. You'll have more energy, you'll feel healthy, you'll hardly ever get sick again and you'll bounce out of bed in the morning with less than 8 hours of sleep!

We could list 1000 things that work or don't work for losing weight, but cutting out excuses, sugar, starchy carbs and food additives cover about 95% of weight loss "secrets". The rest is up to you. It's a journey, a fun one. A journey tailored only for you.

**You're an athlete now. Athletes experiment.**

If you read about food secrets in a magazine and want to try them, don't just believe the marketing hype, experiment on yourself first. Remember that you are unique. What works for you might not work for us and vice versa. Be scientific about it! Change one thing at a time, and observe.

For example, you may have heard that wheat is harmful to you and you'd like to find out if it is. For one week then, do everything exactly the same as last week, except cut out wheat.

By the end of the week, you'll be able to tell if you have wheat intolerance. If you do, you will feel so good having not had any that you will never want to eat it again. If you don't have intolerance to wheat, you will feel no different.

Losing the winter coat and becoming the athlete underneath is simple. It's simply time to choose it. If you face roadblocks then use Maggie's CPR Mind Potential audios to overcome them and ask for help.

You are an athlete, choose to remember it today.

*Have fun*
*Sharny and Julius*

## Summary

| 12 Steps to Healthy Eating and Perfect Athleticism by Sharny & Julius Kieser | |
|---|---|
| Step 1: | Take Responsibility for what you put in your mouth |
| Step 2: | Change Your Perspective: Never say that you're fat again |
| Step 3: | Realise you are an athlete (a damn powerful one!) |
| Step 4: | Exercise all the muscles in your body to prevent them being eaten |

*(continued)*

| Step 5: | Only exercise for as long as you need in order to move EVERY muscle so that you take your muscles off the menu. Do this for a period of time till you've worked each muscle enthusiastically, only do more if you're enjoying it |
| --- | --- |
| Step 6: | Prevent yourself from ever gaining weight again, *then* work on losing what you've stored |
| Step 7: | Quit Sugar |
| Step 8: | Cheating is for losers. No Cheat Days. You're a winner. |
| Step 9: | Don't fatten up your meals with starch |
| Step 10: | Additives are unpredictable, don't eat numbers |
| Step 11: | Google MSG |
| Step 12: | Food is fuel, not entertainment |

## Maggie Wilde's thoughts:

Well, what can I say to that? Thanks Sharny and Julius for providing your 12 straight talking, guns blazing, easy steps to success. Like they said: don't just take their word for it, approach what they have said scientifically and do your own research. Find out what is right for you because you are unique.

Take one step and apply it to your life each week. If it works for you, you'll feel better. Remember you have the audios and all of the other exercises in my book to help you do this too: Use the CPR – Mind Potential Kit to overcome obstacles, eliminate the sugar and carbohydrate cravings and build motivation, as you program and rewire your mind for success.

## In summary:

Think of yourself as an athlete who has a winter coat of fat to unzip. Ask yourself: *What would an elite athlete choose to eat?*

If you are being honest, it will be something healthy. Take responsibility to do the commitments, eat less and choose smaller portions, take your muscles off the menu and move your muscles more, cut out starch, additives, sugar and blame!

Remember I mentioned raising your adversity quotient in Chapter 6: this simply means when your life is not how you want it to be: stop blaming others, yourself and the world.

Take responsibility for your healthy body and mind, use the audios provided to help you overcome challenges. Drop me a line at info@thepotentialist.com if you need further help.

Be happy, slim and healthy
*Maggie Wilde*

| **Remember your 10 Commitments** |
|:---:|
| Rehearse Outfit |
| Audio Daily |
| Weigh Once |
| Stomach chooses |
| Smaller Portions |
| Chew Slowly |
| Push Plate |
| Thirst = Water |
| Wiggle Move |
| Write Progress |

# FOURTEEN

## Feed the Mind – Progress Journal to Success

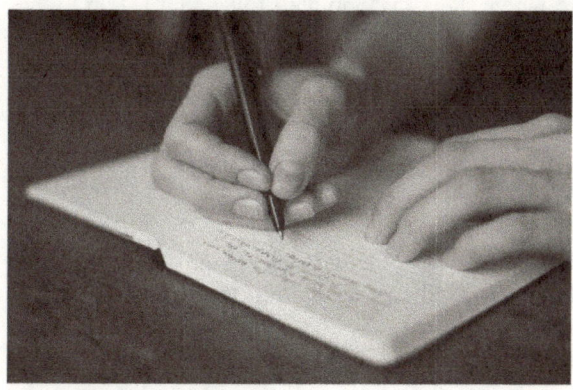

Remember Commitment 10 – Write Progress? Using our Progress Journal to Success?

This journaling system, when used with the CPR audios is the key, of all keys to unzipping the fat suit for good. I promise!

If you've ever used journaling before you'll soon recognise that this journal will ask something a little different of you. If you haven't used journaling, then please read this chapter with an open mind and a willing heart. You've come this far through the book; it's worth trusting in this process too. Once you grasp this journaling system and the reason why it's so important, you will have ALL the keys to change your eating patterns, unzip the fat suit and be slim and healthy permanently.

My whole point in writing this book was to provide you with all the keys and tools you will ever need to control, program and rewire your mind for slim and healthy permanently. This is the key that gels all of the strategies in the book, the CPR audios and the 10 Commitments together.

I recommend using this journal just before you go to sleep each night. One of the reasons for using it before you go to sleep is that your subconscious mind is processing even while you sleep. If the last thing you think about consciously before you sleep is how easy it is to be slim and healthy, or how amazing you look in your goal outfit, or how much you enjoyed being healthy today, then the subconscious will be processing these great and positive concepts and feelings all night.

When you use this system as you go to sleep, your mind will *'marinate'* on the joys of slim and healthy for the following 6 – 8 hours. If you are anything like I used to be, I used to spend those last few minutes mulling over the stress of work, who said what to whom, how disappointed I was that I didn't work out that day and on and on I could go. I'd make hopeful promises that I'd ignore the biscuit barrel tomorrow at morning tea, all the while thinking, at the back of my mind, that I was kidding myself again.

However, when I started putting this system into practice, my habits began to change more easily. I'd wake in the morning looking forward to my walk knowing I would have that proud feeling after I came back. I would smile to myself as I easily and willingly walked past the biscuit barrel or said no to the cakes and sweats on offer at work.

Use the journal just before sleep time and let your mind marinate for the next 6-8 hours on the slim, healthy, motivated you. That's much better than marinating on how crappy the day was, or how hard tomorrow is going to be, or what you wish you'd said to whomever hurt you all those years ago.

Last thing at night is when you want your subconscious to help you; it is when you want it to focus on what you wish to create, rather than what you don't want to happen anymore.

In the morning as you begin the process of waking, there is a moment when you are not quite awake and not quite asleep, it's a drowsy natural state of self-hypnosis called the hypnopompic state. While you are in this state, think about those successful statements you wrote in your journal the night before. Imagine yourself comfortably in your goal outfit or how great it will feel after you finish exercising your body today, or how good it feels to make healthier choices because you want to. Your brain is then more likely to be wired for the success you wanted and how great you will feel.

## Feed Your Mind

In 2010 a colleague named Stuart Walter was working with a professional golfer to help him improve his game. Stuart specialises in the psychology of sports, helping sporting professionals get better at what they do. The golfer mentioned to Stuart that he had been journaling each night. Stuart asked *"Why do you write about what you did that day, it's already history?"*

Stuart hypothesised that if that day had been filled with what the golfer didn't want any more *(bad shots and bad putting)*, then why would he choose to reinforce the 'bad shots' by writing about them. It is a natural process of the mind to imagine and visualise as you write and read while you're doing it. If the mind really doesn't know the difference between real and imagined, then when the golfer's day did not produce what he wanted *(better shots, better putting)*, then his mind was reinforcing and replaying more of what he didn't want *(bad shots, bad putting)*.

If, on the other hand, the golfer wrote about an imagined successful future, a tomorrow filled with everything he wanted to happen, then he would rewire and program his mind with what he wanted the future to be instead. This principle fits perfectly with the fact that 'the mind does not know the difference between real and imagined'. You can imagine the success of tomorrow today, and the brain won't know it isn't real. Your brain will then have a memory (neural pathway) of performing that success. You are more likely to experience the same motivation, energy and actions you imagined in your mind.

## Try this exercise:

**Take a pen and paper and write down the sentence**: *I slammed my finger in the car door.*

What happened when you did that? Did you get an image or impression in your mind of a squashed finger? Did you imagine / feel the flinch? Did your mind provide an image/memory that matched the statement?

**Now write down**: *I loved the walk on the beach today, the water cleansed my feet.*

What happened when you wrote that statement? Did you sense the fantastic energy after a beach walk? Did you imagine or feel how good it would be with the coolness of your feet in the water? Did your mind provide an image or impression/memory that matched the statement? Were you able to imagine or sense what it would feel like to do that?

This is precisely what will happen when you use this journaling process. By writing about something positive that hasn't happened yet, your mind will continue to program and rewire for the desired positive outcome. The foundation of the success 'memories' that you imagine, will be laid down in your brain.

The more you use this technique by writing about the successful things, active things, motivating slim and healthy things you wish to achieve, the more your mind will create the image or impression, and the more it will help stimulate the desire to do the things you wish to do.

## Remember your 'Perception Library' and 'Pharmacist'?

By doing this technique the Library now has a positive perception of waking with energy and enjoying exercise, because you already imagined it as you wrote about it in your journal the night before. It is now more likely to send the positive message to the Pharmacist. The Pharmacist is more likely to activate the Neuro-chemicals that stimulate feeling happier and motivated when you think about moving your body or exercising.

If you write about the healthy choices you made tomorrow as if it is real today, then your mind and brain will create the impression or memory of it and begin to help you produce the physical motivation and action more easily within days too. Remember, according to Dr Leaf's research, your brain begins to rewire healthier neural pathways within days of actively creating more positive thoughts and feelings.

When you practice the art of pretending that tomorrow has already happened successfully, when you do this by writing about it and adding positive sensations and feelings, your brain will release more helpful chemicals to motivate you. You begin to naturally feel good about physically doing these things when tomorrow comes.

This commitment takes us back to two of our original Keys

1. **Real or imagined** - 'Your mind doesn't know the difference between real and imagined, what it sees it believes.'
2. **Imagination** – Mind Rehearsal and how your brain learns and rewires better habits, behaviours, beliefs and feelings.

## Your Progress Journal to Success

Your Progress Journal is no ordinary journal. It's more a *Slim & Healthy Projection* Journal. The journal itself has been adapted from that wonderful technique that Stuart Walter developed while working with the golfer. The technique was so successful that Stuart wrote a book *"The Dear Diary Process"*.

When Stuart gifted me his book, I immediately put it to use and soon realised it was an amazing way to improve my focus in all areas of my life. I adapted it with Stuart's permission and began using it with all of my clients to help them increase focus and momentum to unzip the fat suit and change eating patterns too.

As I have mentioned quite often in this book, when we use mind rehearsal to achieve a new outcome we connect and fire new neural pathways. These neural pathways create a 'memory' in the brain, a circuitry that becomes linked to the sense that the success you are after is already 'known' to you. You then find doing those pre-rehearsed things easier to achieve. It's as though your brain thinks you have already done it, so it simply keeps sending the right communication and Neuro-chemicals to do it again. That's what this process does for you.

By committing to use this system, you can pre-program your brain faster while using the 10 Commitments and CPR audios to think and take action as though the slim and healthy behaviour is normal.

Within a few days of using this Mind Rehearsal Progress Journal you will easily notice the difference. The actions you need to take, the new healthy way you now want to respond to challenges will seem easier to achieve somehow. Synchronicity, ideas, and the help and motivation to achieve your ideal weight, shape and size will be there for you.

**Please note: I have provided a couple of sample Progress Journal entries later to help you understand the process**

## So the steps are easy:

At the end of the day open your journal:

Step 1:   **Write tomorrow's date on the page**

Step 2:   **Write about tomorrow's success in the past tense**. Write in the past tense as if it is has already happened. E.g. "I felt proud after my walk today" or "I was so energised after my walk" or "it felt so good to leave food on the plate and push it away". Remember when you did the exercise earlier about writing the two different statements? *"I slammed my finger in the car door" and "I loved the walk on the beach today, the water cleansed my feet"*. Your mind took you to those places as you wrote. You had a different response to the door slam than you had to the beach walk.

In a traditional journaling process where you write about the day that has just finished, you might write something like: *"I had a bad day today, I couldn't resist the biscuits at work"*. As you write that, your mind would re-experience the biscuits, the disappointment or whatever emotion you experienced during that day. Your subconscious mind would then be marinating as you slept on the heightened emotions attached to 'biscuits', 'temptation' and 'guilt or regret'. Not a recipe for waking with a refreshed attitude and healthy ideas.

On the other hand, using the Unzip the Fat Suit Progress Journal you can program tomorrow for successful healthy actions and thoughts. By writing success projections as if they have already happened, by imagining or pretending those projections, your mind will replay those success emotions and images while you write. Your subconscious will sleep on the great sensations and feelings being healthy and active created for you.

**Step 3: Imagine Using All of Your Senses 'acting out how good it feels'.**

a.    You might write "It felt so good to know I had had enough lunch before I even got half way through it. I remembered to chew more slowly. It felt easier to say 'enough is enough'."

b.    Or you might write "I felt so great after my walk today and I actually wanted to do it too. I am proud of myself for finishing all the commitments today, I enjoyed listening to my audios."

c.    By doing this every night you will be programming your mind for faster results. This process works on the same principles as the CPR audios. It's about giving yourself permission to go with it, pretend, act as if it's happened already. Feel what you feel as if you were actually doing what you are writing about. Allow yourself to *be in it,* and trust the process. Even if you feel silly at first, within a few days, your Progress Journal entries start to come true for you.

Because the mind does not know the difference, you will pre-program tomorrow in your mind tonight. So when tomorrow does come, your mind is more likely to provide the right chemical reaction for more motivation, effortless ability to make healthier choices or whatever it is you have pre-programmed.

Remember: if today is Wednesday 15th then write Thursday 16th on the top of the page and write the successes you achieved Thursday as if it has already happened. Let your imagination take you away to that successful feeling when you achieve these slim and healthy things easily.

The key is to read it back to yourself to allow your mind to absorb the 'feelings' associated with what you have written. How good it felt, how easy it was, how pleased you feel.

**Stuart Walter says, "This is not a 'To Do List' it is a 'Have Done List'."**

Remember write your progress journal to meet your needs and use your own words. Some people focus on areas they have been challenged by in the past. This is achieved by writing success statements about overcoming those challenges daily so that they program and rewire for a better outcome now. Others use images, cutting pictures out of magazines or photos that stimulate them to know how they will feel when this success occurs. Whatever works for you is fine.

I have provided a couple of sample progress journal entries to help you understand how to make this system work best for you. These are examples only; you do not have to use these exact words. Tailor your entries specific to you. I have based these samples on the 10 Commitments and the healthy suggestions within the book and the audios that create the slim and healthy you.

## Sample 1: Unzip the Fat Suit Progress Journal
*(Written Wednesday 18th January - just before bedtime)*

## Day & Date <u>Thursday 19th January</u>

I felt amazing today. It was so much fun to find ways to move my body more, I parked my car 3 blocks from work and walked! I loved feeling motivated to do that. I found myself thinking of my goal outfit spontaneously throughout the day. I imagined how hubby smiled at me when I wore it. I surprised myself when I realised how easy it was to remember to chew slowly, I thought about how small my tummy really is. I remember thinking at lunchtime how much fuller I felt after only three quarters of my lunch. I laughed out loud when I pushed the rest away. It felt good to be in control.

## Sample 2: Unzip the Fat Suit Progress Journal
*Written Thursday 19ᵗʰ January just before bedtime*

## Day & Date <u>Friday 20th January</u>

Wow what a day! I felt so much stronger and in control of my food choices. Today was great, I said no to lollies that Jenny offered me at lunchtime and it felt sooo good to genuinely not want one. I am so proud of myself. On my way home from work I stopped at the supermarket and bought a lean chicken breast for dinner that I had with the crunchiest fresh salad that I can ever remember having, I couldn't even finish it, so I packed the rest in a container for lunch tomorrow. I am so organised. I came out of the shop and realised I had just walked by the chocolate aisle and chocolate didn't even cross my mind. I really think this slim and healthy thing is getting easier by the day.

If you want to add pictures, draw or cut and paste magazine images to highlight certain feelings, or actions throughout the day, please make it as creative a process as you wish to. I had one client who didn't do the 'writing thing'. She would cut out or print off images of the things she imagined she had already done, and make up stories in her head about them.

For example, she would paste a picture of a woman walking on a beach or riding a bike and she would take a moment or two to imagine as if she was that woman. In her head she would act as if she was on the bike, she would think about the wind on her skin as she cycled by, or the muscles in her legs getting stronger each time she rode.

Play with the journal, do what's right for you. If writing is challenging at first, use images like the previous client did. It helped her direct her focus and get into the swing of it. Later she began to write too.

Remember: the more emotion, energy and enthusiasm you put into writing and re-reading it, the more the brain will develop those new neural pathways.

To get you started I have provided your first month's Progress Journal. Your thinking and behaviour will begin to adjust to the 10 Commitments even within the first few days when you use this process and the CPR Mind Potential audios. I've been journaling this way for a few years now and even after all this time; I map my success in all areas of my life with this process.

I wish you well on your journaling progress. I wish you joy on your unzip the fat suit journey, and I wish you health and happiness always.

Remember, you have a wealth of strategies, tools and audios to help you on your unzip the fat suit path to slim and healthy. I can't force you to use them, however I can promise you:

Once you start to use them, within a few days you will *choose* to use them more and more, and when you do: the fat suit will begin to fall away.

There are no excuses to stay in the fat suit anymore because:

**Here's a reminder of all the jewels you now have to Unzip the Fat Suit, Control, Program and Rewire your Mind & Body to think and be slim and healthy permanently:**

## Summary of Strategies and Solutions to Use

- The 10 Commitments: Chapter 2
- The 10 Commitments Reminder Summary Chart for the home/car/office
- The CPR-Mind Potential Kit including:
  - Numerous Control (tapping) audios
  - Numerous Program audios
  - Numerous Rewire audios
  - All the exercises and tips in the book
- Numerous Demonstration Videos on YouTube
- 5 Keys to help you think Slim and Healthy: Chapter 1

- 12 + Tips and 2 Questionnaires to recognise, control and eliminate Sabotage/Comfort hungers etc: Chapter 3
- 30 + tips to Control Greedy Appetite Chapter 3
- 14 + Tips on the 'Power of Three List' – To Interrupt & Control Greedy Appetite: Chapter 3 & 4
- 4 x Control & Conquer Audios
- Craving Buster Cheat Sheet to control cravings/feelings: Chapter 4
- Short Cheat Sheet to control cravings/feelings: Chapter 4
- 6 + Belief Audit Tips: 'Ask, Answer, Discuss' questions in Chapters 5
- Control Unhelpful Thinking: Inner Critic versus Inner Coach: Chapter 5
- 6 + Control Unhelpful Thinking Tips: 'Ask/Answer/Discuss': Chapter 5
- 6 + Control Unhelpful Emotional States Tips: Chapter 5
- 6 + Control Unhelpful Behaviour Tips: 'Ask, Answer, Discuss': Chapter 5
- Change Unhelpful Thinking Chart Chapter 5
- 10 + Disconnect Emotions & Food Exercises & Tips: Chapter 6
- Private Investigator Gauge: The P.I.G. Question: *Is this mouthful satisfying nutritional, habitual or my emotional needs?*
- I AM list: Chapter 7
- 8+ Rewire Your Inner Image – Self Confidence Exercises: Chapter 7
- Rewire Build Confidence audios
- 5 + Tips to Rewire Digestion for Slim & Healthy: Chapter 8
- 8 + Tips to increase motivation to exercise and move your body: Chapter 9
- Exercise Mantra: "I'm the kind of person who enjoys moving my body": Chapter 9
- Motivation to Move Your Body & Exercise Program Audio
- Letting go of excuses Tips: Chapter 9
- Rewire Slim and Healthy audios
- 30 + Program Metabolism Tips: Chapter 10
- 6 + Once it's off – Keep it off Tips: Chapter 11
- Numerous 'I Can Do It' - Once it's off – Keep it off Control audios
- 30 + Rewire Stress Tips: Chapter 12
- Rewire Nutrition & Athleticism: (Sharny & Julius' 12 Step Process): Chapter 13
- The Inner Athlete mantra: *"What would a slim and healthy athlete eat?"*: Chapter 13
- Progress Journal To Success (Chapter 14)
- Sample Progress Journal entries

Happy days! Remember you can also email me at: info@thepotentialist.com too and check out our Unzip the Fat Suit workshop schedule and online webinars.

N.B. There are also numerous other support audios available for purchase on my website if you wish: www.thepotentialist.com

## Examples include:

- Release Anger & Resentment
- Stop Self Sabotage
- Travelator to Emotional Balance, Health & Wellbeing
- Tone and Firm from the Inside: Hypnosis Liposuction
- Mind Mirror – Create Your Ideal Weight, Shape & Size
- Immune System Support
- Hypnosis Gastric Band 1 & 2

And others…

Each audio can be used separately or added to the Mind Potential: Unzip the Fat Suit Program too.

Wishing you lifelong health and happiness and slim and healthy dreams!

With love from
*Maggie Wilde*

# PROGRESS JOURNAL

**Day & Date** _____

I completed my Ten Commitments today

| ❏ **MIND REHEARSE GOAL OUFIT** I used mind rehearsal to imagine I can already wear my new Goal Outfit comfortably. | ❏ **AUDIO DAILY** I used my Program &/or Rewire Audio. When I needed to, I used my Control audio to stop cravings. | ❏ **WEIGH ONCE** I have only weighed myself once this week. | ❏ **STOMACH CHOOSES** I consulted my Stomach when I needed food. I chose the healthiest option based on what my stomach felt 'light' about. | ❏ **SMALLER PORTIONS** I served Smaller Portions, I used a smaller plate, I focused on the food on the plate as it disappeared. |
|---|---|---|---|---|
| ❏ **CHEW SLOWLY** I Chewed Slowly. I paused between mouthfuls. I put my knife/fork/food down between bites. I noticed the textures & flavours. I focused on and didn't get distracted by TV or the computer while I ate. | ❏ **PUSH PLATE** I listened/ tuned into my stomach between mouth-fuls and when I knew *Enough was Enough, I* Pushed the Plate away even if there was food still on it. | ❏ **THIRST – WATER** I drank at least 2 litres of water today. I love cleansing my body this way. | ❏ **WIGGLE MOVE** I moved my body more; I put more energy into my movement. I exer-cised in some way. I walked, swam or jogged, I danced or parked further away from the office/ supermarket, I worked out etc. | ❏ **WRITE PROGRESS** I wrote/drew in my Progress journal and enjoyed feeling how easy it is to unzip the fat suit from now on. I can do this. I imagined how easy all the commitments are. |

_____

_____

_____

_____

_____

_____

_____

_____

_____

_____

# PROGRESS JOURNAL

**Day & Date** _____

I completed my Ten Commitments today

| ❑ **MIND REHEARSE GOAL OUFIT** | ❑ **AUDIO DAILY** | ❑ **WEIGH ONCE** | ❑ **STOMACH CHOOSES** | ❑ **SMALLER PORTIONS** |
|---|---|---|---|---|
| I used mind rehearsal to imagine I can already wear my new Goal Outfit comfortably. | I used my Program &/or Rewire Audio. When I needed to, I used my Control audio to stop cravings. | I have only weighed myself once this week. | I consulted my Stomach when I needed food. I chose the healthiest option based on what my stomach felt 'light' about. | I served Smaller Portions, I used a smaller plate, I focused on the food on the plate as it disappeared. |
| ❑ **CHEW SLOWLY** | ❑ **PUSH PLATE** | ❑ **THIRST – WATER** | ❑ **WIGGLE MOVE** | ❑ **WRITE PROGRESS** |
| I Chewed Slowly. I paused between mouthfuls. I put my knife/fork/food down between bites. I noticed the textures & flavours. I focused on and didn't get distracted by TV or the computer while I ate. | I listened/ tuned into my stomach between mouthfuls and when I knew *Enough was Enough, I* Pushed the Plate away even if there was food still on it. | I drank at least 2 litres of water today. I love cleansing my body this way. | I moved my body more; I put more energy into my movement. I exercised in some way. I walked, swam or jogged, I danced or parked further away from the office/ supermarket, I worked out etc. | I wrote/drew in my Progress journal and enjoyed feeling how easy it is to unzip the fat suit from now on. I can do this. I imagined how easy all the commitments are. |

_____

_____

_____

_____

_____

_____

_____

_____

_____

_____

# PROGRESS JOURNAL

**Day & Date** _____

I completed my Ten Commitments today

| ❑ MIND REHEARSE GOAL OUFIT | ❑ AUDIO DAILY | ❑ WEIGH ONCE | ❑ STOMACH CHOOSES | ❑ SMALLER PORTIONS |
|---|---|---|---|---|
| I used mind rehearsal to imagine I can already wear my new Goal Outfit comfortably. | I used my Program &/or Rewire Audio. When I needed to, I used my Control audio to stop cravings. | I have only weighed myself once this week. | I consulted my Stomach when I needed food. I chose the healthiest option based on what my stomach felt 'light' about. | I served Smaller Portions, I used a smaller plate, I focused on the food on the plate as it disappeared. |
| ❑ CHEW SLOWLY | ❑ PUSH PLATE | ❑ THIRST – WATER | ❑ WIGGLE MOVE | ❑ WRITE PROGRESS |
| I Chewed Slowly. I paused between mouthfuls. I put my knife/fork/food down between bites. I noticed the textures & flavours. I focused on and didn't get distracted by TV or the computer while I ate. | I listened/ tuned into my stomach between mouth-fuls and when I knew *Enough was Enough, I* Pushed the Plate away even if there was food still on it. | I drank at least 2 litres of water today. I love cleansing my body this way. | I moved my body more; I put more energy into my movement. I exer-cised in some way. I walked, swam or jogged, I danced or parked further away from the office/ supermarket, I worked out etc. | I wrote/drew in my Progress journal and enjoyed feeling how easy it is to unzip the fat suit from now on. I can do this. I imagined how easy all the commitments are. |

_____

_____

_____

_____

_____

_____

_____

_____

_____

_____

# PROGRESS JOURNAL

**Day & Date** _____

I completed my Ten Commitments today

| ❑ **MIND REHEARSE GOAL OUFIT** | ❑ **AUDIO DAILY** | ❑ **WEIGH ONCE** | ❑ **STOMACH CHOOSES** | ❑ **SMALLER PORTIONS** |
|---|---|---|---|---|
| I used mind rehearsal to imagine I can already wear my new Goal Outfit comfortably. | I used my Program &/or Rewire Audio. When I needed to, I used my Control audio to stop cravings. | I have only weighed myself once this week. | I consulted my Stomach when I needed food. I chose the healthiest option based on what my stomach felt 'light' about. | I served Smaller Portions, I used a smaller plate, I focused on the food on the plate as it disappeared. |
| ❑ **CHEW SLOWLY** | ❑ **PUSH PLATE** | ❑ **THIRST – WATER** | ❑ **WIGGLE MOVE** | ❑ **WRITE PROGRESS** |
| I Chewed Slowly. I paused between mouthfuls. I put my knife/fork/food down between bites. I noticed the textures & flavours. I focused on and didn't get distracted by TV or the computer while I ate. | I listened/ tuned into my stomach between mouthfuls and when I knew *Enough was Enough, I* Pushed the Plate away even if there was food still on it. | I drank at least 2 litres of water today. I love cleansing my body this way. | I moved my body more; I put more energy into my movement. I exercised in some way. I walked, swam or jogged, I danced or parked further away from the office/ supermarket, I worked out etc. | I wrote/drew in my Progress journal and enjoyed feeling how easy it is to unzip the fat suit from now on. I can do this. I imagined how easy all the commitments are. |

_____

_____

_____

_____

_____

_____

_____

_____

_____

_____

# PROGRESS JOURNAL

**Day & Date** _____

I completed my Ten Commitments today

| ❑ MIND REHEARSE GOAL OUFIT | ❑ AUDIO DAILY | ❑ WEIGH ONCE | ❑ STOMACH CHOOSES | ❑ SMALLER PORTIONS |
|---|---|---|---|---|
| I used mind rehearsal to imagine I can already wear my new Goal Outfit comfortably. | I used my Program &/or Rewire Audio. When I needed to, I used my Control audio to stop cravings. | I have only weighed myself once this week. | I consulted my Stomach when I needed food. I chose the healthiest option based on what my stomach felt 'light' about. | I served Smaller Portions, I used a smaller plate, I focused on the food on the plate as it disappeared. |
| ❑ CHEW SLOWLY | ❑ PUSH PLATE | ❑ THIRST – WATER | ❑ WIGGLE MOVE | ❑ WRITE PROGRESS |
| I Chewed Slowly. I paused between mouthfuls. I put my knife/fork/food down between bites. I noticed the textures & flavours. I focused on and didn't get distracted by TV or the computer while I ate. | I listened/ tuned into my stomach between mouth-fuls and when I knew *Enough was Enough, I* Pushed the Plate away even if there was food still on it. | I drank at least 2 litres of water today. I love cleansing my body this way. | I moved my body more; I put more energy into my movement. I exer-cised in some way. I walked, swam or jogged, I danced or parked further away from the office/ supermarket, I worked out etc. | I wrote/drew in my Progress journal and enjoyed feeling how easy it is to unzip the fat suit from now on. I can do this. I imagined how easy all the commitments are. |

_____

_____

_____

_____

_____

_____

_____

_____

_____

_____

# PROGRESS JOURNAL

**Day & Date** _____

I completed my Ten Commitments today

| | | | | |
|---|---|---|---|---|
| ❏ **MIND REHEARSE GOAL OUFIT** I used mind rehearsal to imagine I can already wear my new Goal Outfit comfortably. | ❏ **AUDIO DAILY** I used my Program &/or Rewire Audio. When I needed to, I used my Control audio to stop cravings. | ❏ **WEIGH ONCE** I have only weighed myself once this week. | ❏ **STOMACH CHOOSES** I consulted my Stomach when I needed food. I chose the healthiest option based on what my stomach felt 'light' about. | ❏ **SMALLER PORTIONS** I served Smaller Portions, I used a smaller plate, I focused on the food on the plate as it disappeared. |
| ❏ **CHEW SLOWLY** I Chewed Slowly. I paused between mouthfuls. I put my knife/fork/food down between bites. I noticed the textures & flavours. I focused on and didn't get distracted by TV or the computer while I ate. | ❏ **PUSH PLATE** I listened/ tuned into my stomach between mouth-fuls and when I knew *Enough was Enough*, I Pushed the Plate away even if there was food still on it. | ❏ **THIRST – WATER** I drank at least 2 litres of water today. I love cleansing my body this way. | ❏ **WIGGLE MOVE** I moved my body more; I put more energy into my movement. I exer-cised in some way. I walked, swam or jogged, I danced or parked further away from the office/ supermarket, I worked out etc. | ❏ **WRITE PROGRESS** I wrote/drew in my Progress journal and enjoyed feeling how easy it is to unzip the fat suit from now on. I can do this. I imagined how easy all the commitments are. |

_____

_____

_____

_____

_____

_____

_____

_____

_____

_____

# PROGRESS JOURNAL

**Day & Date** _____

I completed my Ten Commitments today

| ❑ MIND REHEARSE GOAL OUFIT<br>I used mind rehearsal to imagine I can already wear my new Goal Outfit comfortably. | ❑ AUDIO DAILY<br>I used my Program &/or Rewire Audio. When I needed to, I used my Control audio to stop cravings. | ❑ WEIGH ONCE<br>I have only weighed myself once this week. | ❑ STOMACH CHOOSES<br>I consulted my Stomach when I needed food. I chose the healthiest option based on what my stomach felt 'light' about. | ❑ SMALLER PORTIONS<br>I served Smaller Portions, I used a smaller plate, I focused on the food on the plate as it disappeared. |
|---|---|---|---|---|
| ❑ CHEW SLOWLY<br>I Chewed Slowly. I paused between mouthfuls. I put my knife/fork/food down between bites. I noticed the textures & flavours. I focused on and didn't get distracted by TV or the computer while I ate. | ❑ PUSH PLATE<br>I listened/ tuned into my stomach between mouthfuls and when I knew *Enough was Enough, I* Pushed the Plate away even if there was food still on it. | ❑ THIRST – WATER<br>I drank at least 2 litres of water today. I love cleansing my body this way. | ❑ WIGGLE MOVE<br>I moved my body more; I put more energy into my movement. I exercised in some way. I walked, swam or jogged, I danced or parked further away from the office/ supermarket, I worked out etc. | ❑ WRITE PROGRESS<br>I wrote/drew in my Progress journal and enjoyed feeling how easy it is to unzip the fat suit from now on. I can do this. I imagined how easy all the commitments are. |

_____

_____

_____

_____

_____

_____

_____

_____

_____

_____

# PROGRESS JOURNAL

**Day & Date** _____

I completed my Ten Commitments today

| ❏ MIND REHEARSE GOAL OUFIT I used mind rehearsal to imagine I can already wear my new Goal Outfit comfortably. | ❏ AUDIO DAILY I used my Program &/or Rewire Audio. When I needed to, I used my Control audio to stop cravings. | ❏ WEIGH ONCE I have only weighed myself once this week. | ❏ STOMACH CHOOSES I consulted my Stomach when I needed food. I chose the healthiest option based on what my stomach felt 'light' about. | ❏ SMALLER PORTIONS I served Smaller Portions, I used a smaller plate, I focused on the food on the plate as it disappeared. |
|---|---|---|---|---|
| ❏ CHEW SLOWLY I Chewed Slowly. I paused between mouthfuls. I put my knife/fork/food down between bites. I noticed the textures & flavours. I focused on and didn't get distracted by TV or the computer while I ate. | ❏ PUSH PLATE I listened/ tuned into my stomach between mouthfuls and when I knew *Enough was Enough, I* Pushed the Plate away even if there was food still on it. | ❏ THIRST – WATER I drank at least 2 litres of water today. I love cleansing my body this way. | ❏ WIGGLE MOVE I moved my body more; I put more energy into my movement. I exercised in some way. I walked, swam or jogged, I danced or parked further away from the office/ supermarket, I worked out etc. | ❏ WRITE PROGRESS I wrote/drew in my Progress journal and enjoyed feeling how easy it is to unzip the fat suit from now on. I can do this. I imagined how easy all the commitments are. |

_____

_____

_____

_____

_____

_____

_____

_____

_____

_____

_____

# PROGRESS JOURNAL

**Day & Date** _____

I completed my Ten Commitments today

| ❏ MIND REHEARSE GOAL OUFIT | ❏ AUDIO DAILY | ❏ WEIGH ONCE | ❏ STOMACH CHOOSES | ❏ SMALLER PORTIONS |
|---|---|---|---|---|
| I used mind rehearsal to imagine I can already wear my new Goal Outfit comfortably. | I used my Program &/or Rewire Audio. When I needed to, I used my Control audio to stop cravings. | I have only weighed myself once this week. | I consulted my Stomach when I needed food. I chose the healthiest option based on what my stomach felt 'light' about. | I served Smaller Portions, I used a smaller plate, I focused on the food on the plate as it disappeared. |
| ❏ CHEW SLOWLY | ❏ PUSH PLATE | ❏ THIRST – WATER | ❏ WIGGLE MOVE | ❏ WRITE PROGRESS |
| I Chewed Slowly. I paused between mouthfuls. I put my knife/fork/food down between bites. I noticed the textures & flavours. I focused on and didn't get distracted by TV or the computer while I ate. | I listened/ tuned into my stomach between mouthfuls and when I knew *Enough was Enough, I* Pushed the Plate away even if there was food still on it. | I drank at least 2 litres of water today. I love cleansing my body this way. | I moved my body more; I put more energy into my movement. I exercised in some way. I walked, swam or jogged, I danced or parked further away from the office/ supermarket, I worked out etc. | I wrote/drew in my Progress journal and enjoyed feeling how easy it is to unzip the fat suit from now on. I can do this. I imagined how easy all the commitments are. |

_____

_____

_____

_____

_____

_____

_____

_____

_____

_____

_____

# PROGRESS JOURNAL

**Day & Date** _____

I completed my Ten Commitments today

| ❑ MIND REHEARSE GOAL OUFIT I used mind rehearsal to imagine I can already wear my new Goal Outfit comfortably. | ❑ AUDIO DAILY I used my Program &/or Rewire Audio. When I needed to, I used my Control audio to stop cravings. | ❑ WEIGH ONCE I have only weighed myself once this week. | ❑ STOMACH CHOOSES I consulted my Stomach when I needed food. I chose the healthiest option based on what my stomach felt 'light' about. | ❑ SMALLER PORTIONS I served Smaller Portions, I used a smaller plate, I focused on the food on the plate as it disappeared. |
|---|---|---|---|---|
| ❑ CHEW SLOWLY I Chewed Slowly. I paused between mouthfuls. I put my knife/fork/food down between bites. I noticed the textures & flavours. I focused on and didn't get distracted by TV or the computer while I ate. | ❑ PUSH PLATE I listened/ tuned into my stomach between mouth-fuls and when I knew *Enough was Enough, I* Pushed the Plate away even if there was food still on it. | ❑ THIRST – WATER I drank at least 2 litres of water today. I love cleansing my body this way. | ❑ WIGGLE MOVE I moved my body more; I put more energy into my movement. I exer-cised in some way. I walked, swam or jogged, I danced or parked further away from the office/ supermarket, I worked out etc. | ❑ WRITE PROGRESS I wrote/drew in my Progress journal and enjoyed feeling how easy it is to unzip the fat suit from now on. I can do this. I imagined how easy all the commitments are. |

_____

_____

_____

_____

_____

_____

_____

_____

_____

# PROGRESS JOURNAL

**Day & Date** _____

I completed my Ten Commitments today

| ❏ MIND REHEARSE GOAL OUFIT | ❏ AUDIO DAILY | ❏ WEIGH ONCE | ❏ STOMACH CHOOSES | ❏ SMALLER PORTIONS |
|---|---|---|---|---|
| I used mind rehearsal to imagine I can already wear my new Goal Outfit comfortably. | I used my Program &/or Rewire Audio. When I needed to, I used my Control audio to stop cravings. | I have only weighed myself once this week. | I consulted my Stomach when I needed food. I chose the healthiest option based on what my stomach felt 'light' about. | I served Smaller Portions, I used a smaller plate, I focused on the food on the plate as it disappeared. |
| **❏ CHEW SLOWLY** | **❏ PUSH PLATE** | **❏ THIRST – WATER** | **❏ WIGGLE MOVE** | **❏ WRITE PROGRESS** |
| I Chewed Slowly. I paused between mouthfuls. I put my knife/fork/food down between bites. I noticed the textures & flavours. I focused on and didn't get distracted by TV or the computer while I ate. | I listened/ tuned into my stomach between mouthfuls and when I knew *Enough was Enough, I* Pushed the Plate away even if there was food still on it. | I drank at least 2 litres of water today. I love cleansing my body this way. | I moved my body more; I put more energy into my movement. I exercised in some way. I walked, swam or jogged, I danced or parked further away from the office/ supermarket, I worked out etc. | I wrote/drew in my Progress journal and enjoyed feeling how easy it is to unzip the fat suit from now on. I can do this. I imagined how easy all the commitments are. |

_____

_____

_____

_____

_____

_____

_____

_____

_____

_____

# PROGRESS JOURNAL

**Day & Date** _____

I completed my Ten Commitments today

| ❏ MIND REHEARSE GOAL OUFIT<br>I used mind rehearsal to imagine I can already wear my new Goal Outfit comfortably. | ❏ AUDIO DAILY<br>I used my Program &/or Rewire Audio. When I needed to, I used my Control audio to stop cravings. | ❏ WEIGH ONCE<br>I have only weighed myself once this week. | ❏ STOMACH CHOOSES<br>I consulted my Stomach when I needed food. I chose the healthiest option based on what my stomach felt 'light' about. | ❏ SMALLER PORTIONS<br>I served Smaller Portions, I used a smaller plate, I focused on the food on the plate as it disappeared. |
|---|---|---|---|---|
| ❏ CHEW SLOWLY<br>I Chewed Slowly. I paused between mouthfuls. I put my knife/fork/food down between bites. I noticed the textures & flavours. I focused on and didn't get distracted by TV or the computer while I ate. | ❏ PUSH PLATE<br>I listened/ tuned into my stomach between mouthfuls and when I knew *Enough was Enough, I* Pushed the Plate away even if there was food still on it. | ❏ THIRST – WATER<br>I drank at least 2 litres of water today. I love cleansing my body this way. | ❏ WIGGLE MOVE<br>I moved my body more; I put more energy into my movement. I exercised in some way. I walked, swam or jogged, I danced or parked further away from the office/ supermarket, I worked out etc. | ❏ WRITE PROGRESS<br>I wrote/drew in my Progress journal and enjoyed feeling how easy it is to unzip the fat suit from now on. I can do this. I imagined how easy all the commitments are. |

_____

_____

_____

_____

_____

_____

_____

_____

_____

_____

# PROGRESS JOURNAL

**Day & Date** _____

I completed my Ten Commitments today

| ❏ **MIND REHEARSE GOAL OUFIT** I used mind rehearsal to imagine I can already wear my new Goal Outfit comfortably. | ❏ **AUDIO DAILY** I used my Program &/or Rewire Audio. When I needed to, I used my Control audio to stop cravings. | ❏ **WEIGH ONCE** I have only weighed myself once this week. | ❏ **STOMACH CHOOSES** I consulted my Stomach when I needed food. I chose the healthiest option based on what my stomach felt 'light' about. | ❏ **SMALLER PORTIONS** I served Smaller Portions, I used a smaller plate, I focused on the food on the plate as it disappeared. |
| --- | --- | --- | --- | --- |
| ❏ **CHEW SLOWLY** I Chewed Slowly. I paused between mouthfuls. I put my knife/fork/food down between bites. I noticed the textures & flavours. I focused on and didn't get distracted by TV or the computer while I ate. | ❏ **PUSH PLATE** I listened/ tuned into my stomach between mouth-fuls and when I knew *Enough was Enough, I* Pushed the Plate away even if there was food still on it. | ❏ **THIRST – WATER** I drank at least 2 litres of water today. I love cleansing my body this way. | ❏ **WIGGLE MOVE** I moved my body more; I put more energy into my movement. I exercised in some way. I walked, swam or jogged, I danced or parked further away from the office/ supermarket, I worked out etc. | ❏ **WRITE PROGRESS** I wrote/drew in my Progress journal and enjoyed feeling how easy it is to unzip the fat suit from now on. I can do this. I imagined how easy all the commitments are. |

_____

_____

_____

_____

_____

_____

_____

_____

_____

_____

# PROGRESS JOURNAL

**Day & Date** _____

I completed my Ten Commitments today

| ❑ MIND REHEARSE GOAL OUFIT | ❑ AUDIO DAILY | ❑ WEIGH ONCE | ❑ STOMACH CHOOSES | ❑ SMALLER PORTIONS |
|---|---|---|---|---|
| I used mind rehearsal to imagine I can already wear my new Goal Outfit comfortably. | I used my Program &/or Rewire Audio. When I needed to, I used my Control audio to stop cravings. | I have only weighed myself once this week. | I consulted my Stomach when I needed food. I chose the healthiest option based on what my stomach felt 'light' about. | I served Smaller Portions, I used a smaller plate, I focused on the food on the plate as it disappeared. |
| ❑ CHEW SLOWLY | ❑ PUSH PLATE | ❑ THIRST – WATER | ❑ WIGGLE MOVE | ❑ WRITE PROGRESS |
| I Chewed Slowly. I paused between mouthfuls. I put my knife/fork/food down between bites. I noticed the textures & flavours. I focused on and didn't get distracted by TV or the computer while I ate. | I listened/ tuned into my stomach between mouth-fuls and when I knew *Enough was Enough, I* Pushed the Plate away even if there was food still on it. | I drank at least 2 litres of water today. I love cleansing my body this way. | I moved my body more; I put more energy into my movement. I exercised in some way. I walked, swam or jogged, I danced or parked further away from the office/ supermarket, I worked out etc. | I wrote/drew in my Progress journal and enjoyed feeling how easy it is to unzip the fat suit from now on. I can do this. I imagined how easy all the commitments are. |

_____

_____

_____

_____

_____

_____

_____

_____

_____

_____

# PROGRESS JOURNAL

**Day & Date** _____

I completed my Ten Commitments today

| ❑ **MIND REHEARSE GOAL OUFIT** I used mind rehearsal to imagine I can already wear my new Goal Outfit comfortably. | ❑ **AUDIO DAILY** I used my Program &/or Rewire Audio. When I needed to, I used my Control audio to stop cravings. | ❑ **WEIGH ONCE** I have only weighed myself once this week. | ❑ **STOMACH CHOOSES** I consulted my Stomach when I needed food. I chose the healthiest option based on what my stomach felt 'light' about. | ❑ **SMALLER PORTIONS** I served Smaller Portions, I used a smaller plate, I focused on the food on the plate as it disappeared. |
|---|---|---|---|---|
| ❑ **CHEW SLOWLY** I Chewed Slowly. I paused between mouthfuls. I put my knife/fork/food down between bites. I noticed the textures & flavours. I focused on and didn't get distracted by TV or the computer while I ate. | ❑ **PUSH PLATE** I listened/ tuned into my stomach between mouth-fuls and when I knew *Enough was Enough, I* Pushed the Plate away even if there was food still on it. | ❑ **THIRST – WATER** I drank at least 2 litres of water today. I love cleansing my body this way. | ❑ **WIGGLE MOVE** I moved my body more; I put more energy into my movement. I exer-cised in some way. I walked, swam or jogged, I danced or parked further away from the office/ supermarket, I worked out etc. | ❑ **WRITE PROGRESS** I wrote/drew in my Progress journal and enjoyed feeling how easy it is to unzip the fat suit from now on. I can do this. I imagined how easy all the commitments are. |

_____

_____

_____

_____

_____

_____

_____

_____

_____

_____

_____

# PROGRESS JOURNAL

**Day & Date** _____

I completed my Ten Commitments today

| ❑ **MIND REHEARSE GOAL OUFIT** I used mind rehearsal to imagine I can already wear my new Goal Outfit comfortably. | ❑ **AUDIO DAILY** I used my Program &/or Rewire Audio. When I needed to, I used my Control audio to stop cravings. | ❑ **WEIGH ONCE** I have only weighed myself once this week. | ❑ **STOMACH CHOOSES** I consulted my Stomach when I needed food. I chose the healthiest option based on what my stomach felt 'light' about. | ❑ **SMALLER PORTIONS** I served Smaller Portions, I used a smaller plate, I focused on the food on the plate as it disappeared. |
|---|---|---|---|---|
| ❑ **CHEW SLOWLY** I Chewed Slowly. I paused between mouthfuls. I put my knife/fork/food down between bites. I noticed the textures & flavours. I focused on and didn't get distracted by TV or the computer while I ate. | ❑ **PUSH PLATE** I listened/ tuned into my stomach between mouthfuls and when I knew *Enough was Enough, I* Pushed the Plate away even if there was food still on it. | ❑ **THIRST – WATER** I drank at least 2 litres of water today. I love cleansing my body this way. | ❑ **WIGGLE MOVE** I moved my body more; I put more energy into my movement. I exercised in some way. I walked, swam or jogged, I danced or parked further away from the office/ supermarket, I worked out etc. | ❑ **WRITE PROGRESS** I wrote/drew in my Progress journal and enjoyed feeling how easy it is to unzip the fat suit from now on. I can do this. I imagined how easy all the commitments are. |

_____

_____

_____

_____

_____

_____

_____

_____

_____

# PROGRESS JOURNAL

**Day & Date** _____

I completed my Ten Commitments today

| ❑ **MIND REHEARSE GOAL OUFIT** I used mind rehearsal to imagine I can already wear my new Goal Outfit comfortably. | ❑ **AUDIO DAILY** I used my Program &/or Rewire Audio. When I needed to, I used my Control audio to stop cravings. | ❑ **WEIGH ONCE** I have only weighed myself once this week. | ❑ **STOMACH CHOOSES** I consulted my Stomach when I needed food. I chose the healthiest option based on what my stomach felt 'light' about. | ❑ **SMALLER PORTIONS** I served Smaller Portions, I used a smaller plate, I focused on the food on the plate as it disappeared. |
|---|---|---|---|---|
| ❑ **CHEW SLOWLY** I Chewed Slowly. I paused between mouthfuls. I put my knife/fork/food down between bites. I noticed the textures & flavours. I focused on and didn't get distracted by TV or the computer while I ate. | ❑ **PUSH PLATE** I listened/ tuned into my stomach between mouth-fuls and when I knew _Enough was Enough, I_ Pushed the Plate away even if there was food still on it. | ❑ **THIRST – WATER** I drank at least 2 litres of water today. I love cleansing my body this way. | ❑ **WIGGLE MOVE** I moved my body more; I put more energy into my movement. I exer-cised in some way. I walked, swam or jogged, I danced or parked further away from the office/ supermarket, I worked out etc. | ❑ **WRITE PROGRESS** I wrote/drew in my Progress journal and enjoyed feeling how easy it is to unzip the fat suit from now on. I can do this. I imagined how easy all the commitments are. |

_____

_____

_____

_____

_____

_____

_____

_____

_____

_____

# PROGRESS JOURNAL

**Day & Date** _____

I completed my Ten Commitments today

| ❏ MIND REHEARSE GOAL OUFIT | ❏ AUDIO DAILY | ❏ WEIGH ONCE | ❏ STOMACH CHOOSES | ❏ SMALLER PORTIONS |
|---|---|---|---|---|
| I used mind rehearsal to imagine I can already wear my new Goal Outfit comfortably. | I used my Program &/or Rewire Audio. When I needed to, I used my Control audio to stop cravings. | I have only weighed myself once this week. | I consulted my Stomach when I needed food. I chose the healthiest option based on what my stomach felt 'light' about. | I served Smaller Portions, I used a smaller plate, I focused on the food on the plate as it disappeared. |
| ❏ CHEW SLOWLY | ❏ PUSH PLATE | ❏ THIRST – WATER | ❏ WIGGLE MOVE | ❏ WRITE PROGRESS |
| I Chewed Slowly. I paused between mouthfuls. I put my knife/fork/food down between bites. I noticed the textures & flavours. I focused on and didn't get distracted by TV or the computer while I ate. | I listened/ tuned into my stomach between mouthfuls and when I knew *Enough was Enough, I* Pushed the Plate away even if there was food still on it. | I drank at least 2 litres of water today. I love cleansing my body this way. | I moved my body more; I put more energy into my movement. I exercised in some way. I walked, swam or jogged, I danced or parked further away from the office/ supermarket, I worked out etc. | I wrote/drew in my Progress journal and enjoyed feeling how easy it is to unzip the fat suit from now on. I can do this. I imagined how easy all the commitments are. |

_____

_____

_____

_____

_____

_____

_____

_____

_____

_____

_____

# PROGRESS JOURNAL

**Day & Date** _____

I completed my Ten Commitments today

| ❑ **MIND REHEARSE GOAL OUFIT** I used mind rehearsal to imagine I can already wear my new Goal Outfit comfortably. | ❑ **AUDIO DAILY** I used my Program &/or Rewire Audio. When I needed to, I used my Control audio to stop cravings. | ❑ **WEIGH ONCE** I have only weighed myself once this week. | ❑ **STOMACH CHOOSES** I consulted my Stomach when I needed food. I chose the healthiest option based on what my stomach felt 'light' about. | ❑ **SMALLER PORTIONS** I served Smaller Portions, I used a smaller plate, I focused on the food on the plate as it disappeared. |
|---|---|---|---|---|
| ❑ **CHEW SLOWLY** I Chewed Slowly. I paused between mouthfuls. I put my knife/fork/food down between bites. I noticed the textures & flavours. I focused on and didn't get distracted by TV or the computer while I ate. | ❑ **PUSH PLATE** I listened/ tuned into my stomach between mouthfuls and when I knew *Enough was Enough, I* Pushed the Plate away even if there was food still on it. | ❑ **THIRST – WATER** I drank at least 2 litres of water today. I love cleansing my body this way. | ❑ **WIGGLE MOVE** I moved my body more; I put more energy into my movement. I exercised in some way. I walked, swam or jogged, I danced or parked further away from the office/ supermarket, I worked out etc. | ❑ **WRITE PROGRESS** I wrote/drew in my Progress journal and enjoyed feeling how easy it is to unzip the fat suit from now on. I can do this. I imagined how easy all the commitments are. |

_____

_____

_____

_____

_____

_____

_____

_____

_____

_____

_____

# PROGRESS JOURNAL

**Day & Date** _____

I completed my Ten Commitments today

| ❏ **MIND REHEARSE GOAL OUFIT** I used mind rehearsal to imagine I can already wear my new Goal Outfit comfortably. | ❏ **AUDIO DAILY** I used my Program &/or Rewire Audio. When I needed to, I used my Control audio to stop cravings. | ❏ **WEIGH ONCE** I have only weighed myself once this week. | ❏ **STOMACH CHOOSES** I consulted my Stomach when I needed food. I chose the healthiest option based on what my stomach felt 'light' about. | ❏ **SMALLER PORTIONS** I served Smaller Portions, I used a smaller plate, I focused on the food on the plate as it disappeared. |
|---|---|---|---|---|
| ❏ **CHEW SLOWLY** I Chewed Slowly. I paused between mouthfuls. I put my knife/fork/food down between bites. I noticed the textures & flavours. I focused on and didn't get distracted by TV or the computer while I ate. | ❏ **PUSH PLATE** I listened/ tuned into my stomach between mouthfuls and when I knew *Enough was Enough, I* Pushed the Plate away even if there was food still on it. | ❏ **THIRST – WATER** I drank at least 2 litres of water today. I love cleansing my body this way. | ❏ **WIGGLE MOVE** I moved my body more; I put more energy into my movement. I exercised in some way. I walked, swam or jogged, I danced or parked further away from the office/ supermarket, I worked out etc. | ❏ **WRITE PROGRESS** I wrote/drew in my Progress journal and enjoyed feeling how easy it is to unzip the fat suit from now on. I can do this. I imagined how easy all the commitments are. |

_____

_____

_____

_____

_____

_____

_____

_____

_____

_____

_____

# PROGRESS JOURNAL

**Day & Date** _____

I completed my Ten Commitments today

| ❑ **MIND REHEARSE GOAL OUFIT** I used mind rehearsal to imagine I can already wear my new Goal Outfit comfortably. | ❑ **AUDIO DAILY** I used my Program &/or Rewire Audio. When I needed to, I used my Control audio to stop cravings. | ❑ **WEIGH ONCE** I have only weighed myself once this week. | ❑ **STOMACH CHOOSES** I consulted my Stomach when I needed food. I chose the healthiest option based on what my stomach felt 'light' about. | ❑ **SMALLER PORTIONS** I served Smaller Portions, I used a smaller plate, I focused on the food on the plate as it disappeared. |
|---|---|---|---|---|
| ❑ **CHEW SLOWLY** I Chewed Slowly. I paused between mouthfuls. I put my knife/fork/food down between bites. I noticed the textures & flavours. I focused on and didn't get distracted by TV or the computer while I ate. | ❑ **PUSH PLATE** I listened/ tuned into my stomach between mouth-fuls and when I knew *Enough was Enough, I* Pushed the Plate away even if there was food still on it. | ❑ **THIRST – WATER** I drank at least 2 litres of water today. I love cleansing my body this way. | ❑ **WIGGLE MOVE** I moved my body more; I put more energy into my movement. I exer-cised in some way. I walked, swam or jogged, I danced or parked further away from the office/ supermarket, I worked out etc. | ❑ **WRITE PROGRESS** I wrote/drew in my Progress journal and enjoyed feeling how easy it is to unzip the fat suit from now on. I can do this. I imagined how easy all the commitments are. |

_____

_____

_____

_____

_____

_____

_____

_____

_____

_____

_____

# PROGRESS JOURNAL

**Day & Date** _____

I completed my Ten Commitments today

| | | | | |
|---|---|---|---|---|
| ❏ **MIND REHEARSE GOAL OUFIT** I used mind rehearsal to imagine I can already wear my new Goal Outfit comfortably. | ❏ **AUDIO DAILY** I used my Program &/or Rewire Audio. When I needed to, I used my Control audio to stop cravings. | ❏ **WEIGH ONCE** I have only weighed myself once this week. | ❏ **STOMACH CHOOSES** I consulted my Stomach when I needed food. I chose the healthiest option based on what my stomach felt 'light' about. | ❏ **SMALLER PORTIONS** I served Smaller Portions, I used a smaller plate, I focused on the food on the plate as it disappeared. |
| ❏ **CHEW SLOWLY** I Chewed Slowly. I paused between mouthfuls. I put my knife/fork/food down between bites. I noticed the textures & flavours. I focused on and didn't get distracted by TV or the computer while I ate. | ❏ **PUSH PLATE** I listened/ tuned into my stomach between mouthfuls and when I knew *Enough was Enough, I* Pushed the Plate away even if there was food still on it. | ❏ **THIRST – WATER** I drank at least 2 litres of water today. I love cleansing my body this way. | ❏ **WIGGLE MOVE** I moved my body more; I put more energy into my movement. I exercised in some way. I walked, swam or jogged, I danced or parked further away from the office/ supermarket, I worked out etc. | ❏ **WRITE PROGRESS** I wrote/drew in my Progress journal and enjoyed feeling how easy it is to unzip the fat suit from now on. I can do this. I imagined how easy all the commitments are. |

_____

_____

_____

_____

_____

_____

_____

_____

_____

_____

_____

# PROGRESS JOURNAL

**Day & Date** _____

I completed my Ten Commitments today

| ❑ MIND REHEARSE GOAL OUFIT | ❑ AUDIO DAILY | ❑ WEIGH ONCE | ❑ STOMACH CHOOSES | ❑ SMALLER PORTIONS |
|---|---|---|---|---|
| I used mind rehearsal to imagine I can already wear my new Goal Outfit comfortably. | I used my Program &/or Rewire Audio. When I needed to, I used my Control audio to stop cravings. | I have only weighed myself once this week. | I consulted my Stomach when I needed food. I chose the healthiest option based on what my stomach felt 'light' about. | I served Smaller Portions, I used a smaller plate, I focused on the food on the plate as it disappeared. |
| ❑ CHEW SLOWLY | ❑ PUSH PLATE | ❑ THIRST – WATER | ❑ WIGGLE MOVE | ❑ WRITE PROGRESS |
| I Chewed Slowly. I paused between mouthfuls. I put my knife/fork/food down between bites. I noticed the textures & flavours. I focused on and didn't get distracted by TV or the computer while I ate. | I listened/ tuned into my stomach between mouthfuls and when I knew *Enough was Enough, I* Pushed the Plate away even if there was food still on it. | I drank at least 2 litres of water today. I love cleansing my body this way. | I moved my body more; I put more energy into my movement. I exercised in some way. I walked, swam or jogged, I danced or parked further away from the office/ supermarket, I worked out etc. | I wrote/drew in my Progress journal and enjoyed feeling how easy it is to unzip the fat suit from now on. I can do this. I imagined how easy all the commitments are. |

_____

_____

_____

_____

_____

_____

_____

_____

_____

_____

_____

# PROGRESS JOURNAL

**Day & Date** _____

I completed my Ten Commitments today

| ❑ **MIND REHEARSE GOAL OUFIT** I used mind rehearsal to imagine I can already wear my new Goal Outfit comfortably. | ❑ **AUDIO DAILY** I used my Program &/or Rewire Audio. When I needed to, I used my Control audio to stop cravings. | ❑ **WEIGH ONCE** I have only weighed myself once this week. | ❑ **STOMACH CHOOSES** I consulted my Stomach when I needed food. I chose the healthiest option based on what my stomach felt 'light' about. | ❑ **SMALLER PORTIONS** I served Smaller Portions, I used a smaller plate, I focused on the food on the plate as it disappeared. |
|---|---|---|---|---|
| ❑ **CHEW SLOWLY** I Chewed Slowly. I paused between mouthfuls. I put my knife/fork/food down between bites. I noticed the textures & flavours. I focused on and didn't get distracted by TV or the computer while I ate. | ❑ **PUSH PLATE** I listened/ tuned into my stomach between mouthfuls and when I knew *Enough was Enough, I* Pushed the Plate away even if there was food still on it. | ❑ **THIRST – WATER** I drank at least 2 litres of water today. I love cleansing my body this way. | ❑ **WIGGLE MOVE** I moved my body more; I put more energy into my movement. I exercised in some way. I walked, swam or jogged, I danced or parked further away from the office/ supermarket, I worked out etc. | ❑ **WRITE PROGRESS** I wrote/drew in my Progress journal and enjoyed feeling how easy it is to unzip the fat suit from now on. I can do this. I imagined how easy all the commitments are. |

_____

_____

_____

_____

_____

_____

_____

_____

_____

_____

# PROGRESS JOURNAL

**Day & Date** _____

I completed my Ten Commitments today

| ❑ **MIND REHEARSE GOAL OUFIT** | ❑ **AUDIO DAILY** | ❑ **WEIGH ONCE** | ❑ **STOMACH CHOOSES** | ❑ **SMALLER PORTIONS** |
|---|---|---|---|---|
| I used mind rehearsal to imagine I can already wear my new Goal Outfit comfortably. | I used my Program &/or Rewire Audio. When I needed to, I used my Control audio to stop cravings. | I have only weighed myself once this week. | I consulted my Stomach when I needed food. I chose the healthiest option based on what my stomach felt 'light' about. | I served Smaller Portions, I used a smaller plate, I focused on the food on the plate as it disappeared. |
| ❑ **CHEW SLOWLY** | ❑ **PUSH PLATE** | ❑ **THIRST – WATER** | ❑ **WIGGLE MOVE** | ❑ **WRITE PROGRESS** |
| I Chewed Slowly. I paused between mouthfuls. I put my knife/fork/food down between bites. I noticed the textures & flavours. I focused on and didn't get distracted by TV or the computer while I ate. | I listened/ tuned into my stomach between mouth-fuls and when I knew *Enough was Enough, I* Pushed the Plate away even if there was food still on it. | I drank at least 2 litres of water today. I love cleansing my body this way. | I moved my body more; I put more energy into my movement. I exer-cised in some way. I walked, swam or jogged, I danced or parked further away from the office/ supermarket, I worked out etc. | I wrote/drew in my Progress journal and enjoyed feeling how easy it is to unzip the fat suit from now on. I can do this. I imagined how easy all the commitments are. |

_____

_____

_____

_____

_____

_____

_____

_____

_____

_____

_____

_____

# PROGRESS JOURNAL

**Day & Date** _____

I completed my Ten Commitments today

| ❑ **MIND REHEARSE GOAL OUFIT** I used mind rehearsal to imagine I can already wear my new Goal Outfit comfortably. | ❑ **AUDIO DAILY** I used my Program &/or Rewire Audio. When I needed to, I used my Control audio to stop cravings. | ❑ **WEIGH ONCE** I have only weighed myself once this week. | ❑ **STOMACH CHOOSES** I consulted my Stomach when I needed food. I chose the healthiest option based on what my stomach felt 'light' about. | ❑ **SMALLER PORTIONS** I served Smaller Portions, I used a smaller plate, I focused on the food on the plate as it disappeared. |
|---|---|---|---|---|
| ❑ **CHEW SLOWLY** I Chewed Slowly. I paused between mouthfuls. I put my knife/fork/food down between bites. I noticed the textures & flavours. I focused on and didn't get distracted by TV or the computer while I ate. | ❑ **PUSH PLATE** I listened/ tuned into my stomach between mouthfuls and when I knew *Enough was Enough, I* Pushed the Plate away even if there was food still on it. | ❑ **THIRST – WATER** I drank at least 2 litres of water today. I love cleansing my body this way. | ❑ **WIGGLE MOVE** I moved my body more; I put more energy into my movement. I exercised in some way. I walked, swam or jogged, I danced or parked further away from the office/ supermarket, I worked out etc. | ❑ **WRITE PROGRESS** I wrote/drew in my Progress journal and enjoyed feeling how easy it is to unzip the fat suit from now on. I can do this. I imagined how easy all the commitments are. |

_____

_____

_____

_____

_____

_____

_____

_____

_____

_____

# PROGRESS JOURNAL

**Day & Date** _____

I completed my Ten Commitments today

| ❏ **MIND REHEARSE GOAL OUFIT** I used mind rehearsal to imagine I can already wear my new Goal Outfit comfortably. | ❏ **AUDIO DAILY** I used my Program &/or Rewire Audio. When I needed to, I used my Control audio to stop cravings. | ❏ **WEIGH ONCE** I have only weighed myself once this week. | ❏ **STOMACH CHOOSES** I consulted my Stomach when I needed food. I chose the healthiest option based on what my stomach felt 'light' about. | ❏ **SMALLER PORTIONS** I served Smaller Portions, I used a smaller plate, I focused on the food on the plate as it disappeared. |
|---|---|---|---|---|
| ❏ **CHEW SLOWLY** I Chewed Slowly. I paused between mouthfuls. I put my knife/fork/food down between bites. I noticed the textures & flavours. I focused on and didn't get distracted by TV or the computer while I ate. | ❏ **PUSH PLATE** I listened/ tuned into my stomach between mouth-fuls and when I knew *Enough was Enough, I* Pushed the Plate away even if there was food still on it. | ❏ **THIRST – WATER** I drank at least 2 litres of water today. I love cleansing my body this way. | ❏ **WIGGLE MOVE** I moved my body more; I put more energy into my movement. I exer-cised in some way. I walked, swam or jogged, I danced or parked further away from the office/ supermarket, I worked out etc. | ❏ **WRITE PROGRESS** I wrote/drew in my Progress journal and enjoyed feeling how easy it is to unzip the fat suit from now on. I can do this. I imagined how easy all the commitments are. |

_____

_____

_____

_____

_____

_____

_____

_____

_____

_____

# PROGRESS JOURNAL

**Day & Date** _____

I completed my Ten Commitments today

| ❏ **MIND REHEARSE GOAL OUFIT** I used mind rehearsal to imagine I can already wear my new Goal Outfit comfortably. | ❏ **AUDIO DAILY** I used my Program &/or Rewire Audio. When I needed to, I used my Control audio to stop cravings. | ❏ **WEIGH ONCE** I have only weighed myself once this week. | ❏ **STOMACH CHOOSES** I consulted my Stomach when I needed food. I chose the healthiest option based on what my stomach felt 'light' about. | ❏ **SMALLER PORTIONS** I served Smaller Portions, I used a smaller plate, I focused on the food on the plate as it disappeared. |
|---|---|---|---|---|
| ❏ **CHEW SLOWLY** I Chewed Slowly. I paused between mouthfuls. I put my knife/fork/food down between bites. I noticed the textures & flavours. I focused on and didn't get distracted by TV or the computer while I ate. | ❏ **PUSH PLATE** I listened/ tuned into my stomach between mouth-fuls and when I knew *Enough was Enough, I* Pushed the Plate away even if there was food still on it. | ❏ **THIRST – WATER** I drank at least 2 litres of water today. I love cleansing my body this way. | ❏ **WIGGLE MOVE** I moved my body more; I put more energy into my movement. I exer-cised in some way. I walked, swam or jogged, I danced or parked further away from the office/ supermarket, I worked out etc. | ❏ **WRITE PROGRESS** I wrote/drew in my Progress journal and enjoyed feeling how easy it is to unzip the fat suit from now on. I can do this. I imagined how easy all the commitments are. |

_____

_____

_____

_____

_____

_____

_____

_____

_____

_____

# PROGRESS JOURNAL

**Day & Date** _____

I completed my Ten Commitments today

| ❑ **MIND REHEARSE GOAL OUFIT** I used mind rehearsal to imagine I can already wear my new Goal Outfit comfortably. | ❑ **AUDIO DAILY** I used my Program &/or Rewire Audio. When I needed to, I used my Control audio to stop cravings. | ❑ **WEIGH ONCE** I have only weighed myself once this week. | ❑ **STOMACH CHOOSES** I consulted my Stomach when I needed food. I chose the healthiest option based on what my stomach felt 'light' about. | ❑ **SMALLER PORTIONS** I served Smaller Portions, I used a smaller plate, I focused on the food on the plate as it disappeared. |
|---|---|---|---|---|
| ❑ **CHEW SLOWLY** I Chewed Slowly. I paused between mouthfuls. I put my knife/fork/food down between bites. I noticed the textures & flavours. I focused on and didn't get distracted by TV or the computer while I ate. | ❑ **PUSH PLATE** I listened/ tuned into my stomach between mouth-fuls and when I knew *Enough was Enough, I* Pushed the Plate away even if there was food still on it. | ❑ **THIRST – WATER** I drank at least 2 litres of water today. I love cleansing my body this way. | ❑ **WIGGLE MOVE** I moved my body more; I put more energy into my movement. I exer-cised in some way. I walked, swam or jogged, I danced or parked further away from the office/ supermarket, I worked out etc. | ❑ **WRITE PROGRESS** I wrote/drew in my Progress journal and enjoyed feeling how easy it is to unzip the fat suit from now on. I can do this. I imagined how easy all the commitments are. |

_____

_____

_____

_____

_____

_____

_____

_____

_____

_____

# PROGRESS JOURNAL

**Day & Date** _____

I completed my Ten Commitments today

| ❑ MIND REHEARSE GOAL OUFIT | ❑ AUDIO DAILY | ❑ WEIGH ONCE | ❑ STOMACH CHOOSES | ❑ SMALLER PORTIONS |
|---|---|---|---|---|
| I used mind rehearsal to imagine I can already wear my new Goal Outfit comfortably. | I used my Program &/or Rewire Audio. When I needed to, I used my Control audio to stop cravings. | I have only weighed myself once this week. | I consulted my Stomach when I needed food. I chose the healthiest option based on what my stomach felt 'light' about. | I served Smaller Portions, I used a smaller plate, I focused on the food on the plate as it disappeared. |
| ❑ CHEW SLOWLY | ❑ PUSH PLATE | ❑ THIRST – WATER | ❑ WIGGLE MOVE | ❑ WRITE PROGRESS |
| I Chewed Slowly. I paused between mouthfuls. I put my knife/fork/food down between bites. I noticed the textures & flavours. I focused on and didn't get distracted by TV or the computer while I ate. | I listened/ tuned into my stomach between mouthfuls and when I knew *Enough was Enough, I* Pushed the Plate away even if there was food still on it. | I drank at least 2 litres of water today. I love cleansing my body this way. | I moved my body more; I put more energy into my movement. I exercised in some way. I walked, swam or jogged, I danced or parked further away from the office/ supermarket, I worked out etc. | I wrote/drew in my Progress journal and enjoyed feeling how easy it is to unzip the fat suit from now on. I can do this. I imagined how easy all the commitments are. |

_____

_____

_____

_____

_____

_____

_____

_____

_____

_____

# PROGRESS JOURNAL

**Day & Date** _____

I completed my Ten Commitments today

| ❑ MIND REHEARSE GOAL OUFIT | ❑ AUDIO DAILY | ❑ WEIGH ONCE | ❑ STOMACH CHOOSES | ❑ SMALLER PORTIONS |
|---|---|---|---|---|
| I used mind rehearsal to imagine I can already wear my new Goal Outfit comfortably. | I used my Program &/or Rewire Audio. When I needed to, I used my Control audio to stop cravings. | I have only weighed myself once this week. | I consulted my Stomach when I needed food. I chose the healthiest option based on what my stomach felt 'light' about. | I served Smaller Portions, I used a smaller plate, I focused on the food on the plate as it disappeared. |

| ❑ CHEW SLOWLY | ❑ PUSH PLATE | ❑ THIRST – WATER | ❑ WIGGLE MOVE | ❑ WRITE PROGRESS |
|---|---|---|---|---|
| I Chewed Slowly. I paused between mouthfuls. I put my knife/fork/food down between bites. I noticed the textures & flavours. I focused on and didn't get distracted by TV or the computer while I ate. | I listened/ tuned into my stomach between mouthfuls and when I knew *Enough was Enough, I* Pushed the Plate away even if there was food still on it. | I drank at least 2 litres of water today. I love cleansing my body this way. | I moved my body more; I put more energy into my movement. I exercised in some way. I walked, swam or jogged, I danced or parked further away from the office/ supermarket, I worked out etc. | I wrote/drew in my Progress journal and enjoyed feeling how easy it is to unzip the fat suit from now on. I can do this. I imagined how easy all the commitments are. |

_____

_____

_____

_____

_____

_____

_____

_____

_____

_____

# PROGRESS JOURNAL

**Day & Date** _____

I completed my Ten Commitments today

| ❑ **MIND REHEARSE GOAL OUFIT** I used mind rehearsal to imagine I can already wear my new Goal Outfit comfortably. | ❑ **AUDIO DAILY** I used my Program &/or Rewire Audio. When I needed to, I used my Control audio to stop cravings. | ❑ **WEIGH ONCE** I have only weighed myself once this week. | ❑ **STOMACH CHOOSES** I consulted my Stomach when I needed food. I chose the healthiest option based on what my stomach felt 'light' about. | ❑ **SMALLER PORTIONS** I served Smaller Portions, I used a smaller plate, I focused on the food on the plate as it disappeared. |
|---|---|---|---|---|
| ❑ **CHEW SLOWLY** I Chewed Slowly. I paused between mouthfuls. I put my knife/fork/food down between bites. I noticed the textures & flavours. I focused on and didn't get distracted by TV or the computer while I ate. | ❑ **PUSH PLATE** I listened/ tuned into my stomach between mouth-fuls and when I knew *Enough was Enough, I* Pushed the Plate away even if there was food still on it. | ❑ **THIRST – WATER** I drank at least 2 litres of water today. I love cleansing my body this way. | ❑ **WIGGLE MOVE** I moved my body more; I put more energy into my movement. I exer-cised in some way. I walked, swam or jogged, I danced or parked further away from the office/ supermarket, I worked out etc. | ❑ **WRITE PROGRESS** I wrote/drew in my Progress journal and enjoyed feeling how easy it is to unzip the fat suit from now on. I can do this. I imagined how easy all the commitments are. |

_____

_____

_____

_____

_____

_____

_____

_____

_____

_____

_____

# Appendix

## CPR Mind Potential Kit™

You have been guided at different stages throughout the book to use these free audios and tools from the CPR Mind Potential Kit. If you haven't already done so, download the kit from the link below. Create an 'Unzip the Fat Suit' folder on your own computer to save them in. Transfer them if you wish, to any iPhone/iPod, Mp3 or Android device.

## CPR Mind Potential Kit Content List

**Use this link to download the entire kit: *www.thepotentialist.com/cprkit***

## Control Audios

Control Audio 1:     Control & Conquer – Cravings
Control Audio 2:     Control & Conquer - Unhelpful Emotions/Feelings
Control Audio 3:     Control & Conquer - Self-Doubt & the Fear of Yo-Yo Dieting
Control Audio 4:     Control & Conquer - I Believe in Me/Once it's off I Keep it Off
Control Audio 5:     Control & Conquer – Overeating & Bingeing

## Program Audios

Program Audio 1:     Eliminate Greedy Appetite
Program Audio 2:     Motivation to Move your Body & Exercise
Program Audio 3:     Be Stress Fee

## Rewire Audios

Rewire Audio 1:     Rewire for Slim & Healthy Cardio Version - Unzip the Fat Suit

Rewire Audio 2:     Rewire for Slim & Healthy Relax Version – Unzip the Fat Suit

Rewire Audio 3:     Rewire for Confidence Cardio Version - Build Confidence & Self Esteem

Rewire Audio 4:     Rewire for Confidence Relax Version – Build Confidence & Self Esteem

## CPR Mind Potential Kit Other Tools

- Map Your Progress Chart (Commitment 1)
- 10 Commitments Chart & 10 Commitments Reminder
- Power of Three List
- Quick Cheat Sheet 1 (Control Cravings/Feelings Tapping Chart)
- Craving Buster Cheat Sheet 2 (Control Cravings/Feelings Tapping Chart)
- I AM chart

## YouTube Channel: *http://www.youtube.com/MaggieWilde*

Remember, there are *free* demonstration videos available on my YouTube channel. The videos have been designed to help you gain the most from the Control Tapping techniques. Please feel free to subscribe to my *maggiewilde* YouTube channel for all the current and future demonstration videos.

If you wish to discover other useful Program audios that are available for sale on a variety of different topics including weight reduction, health, emotional release, letting go of habits and more, then may I encourage you to visit the website www. thepotentialist.com

# Bibliography, Recommended Reading & Websites

**Assistant Professor, James Hollis**. April 2012. Iowa State University Chewing Research. http://archive.news.iastate.edu/news/2012/apr/chewing

**Paul G Stoltz,** *Adversity Quotient: Turning obstacles into opportunities http://www.adversityadvantage.com/stoltz.html*

**Dr Caroline Leaf**, *Who Switched off My Brain www.drleaf.com*

**Eckart Tolle**, *The Power of Now www.eckarttolle.com*

**Byron Katie**, *The Three Kinds of Business, Who's Business Are You In, The Work & Loving What Is by Byron Katie www.thework.com*
*http://www.byronkatie.com/2006/09/whose_business_are_you_minding.htm*

**Mireille Guiliano**, *French Women Don't Get Fat www.mireilleguiliano.com*

**John J. Ratey, MD**, *Spark, The Revolutionary New Science of Exercise and the Brain*. www.johnratey.com

**Sharny and Julius Kieser**, *Never Diet Again – Escape the Diet Trap Forever* and *FITlosophy 1 – Chasing Physical Perfection in a World of Gluttony* www.sharnyandjulius.com

**Friedman and Taub 1977,** Hypnosis & Biofeedback Research. References: Friedman, H. & Taub, H. (1977). "The Use of Hypnosis and Biofeedback Procedures for Essential Hypertension." International Journal of Clinical and Experimental Hypnosis, 25, 335-347. (2) Friedman, H. & Taub, H. (1978). "A Six Month Follow-up of the Use of Hypnosis and Biofeedback Procedures in Essential Hypertension." American Journal of Clinical Hypnosis, 20, 184-188

**Native American Cherokee Legend, The Two Wolves,** http://www.firstpeople.us/FP-Html-Legends/TwoWolves-Cherokee.html

**Devin Hastings**, The 5-0 Technique www.devinhastings.com

**Deb Shapiro**, *Your Body Speaks Your Mind, Decoding the Emotional, Psychological and Spiritual Messages that Underlie Illness.* www.debshapiro.com

**Stuart Walter**, The Dear Diary Process. www.athletessecretweapon.com

**Richard Restak, MD**, Brain Rehearsal Research. *The New Brain*, p. 179. PA: Rodale, 2003

**Professor Richard Wiseman**, *59 Seconds – Think a Little Change a Lot.* *http://richardwiseman.wordpress.com/books/*

**Brian Wansink, Ph.D.**, Cornell University http://www.mindlesseating.org/

**Stonyfield Chart,** http://www.stonyfield.com
www.realage.com
Three Magic Words by U.S. Anderson
Iowa State University Chewing Research. http://archive.news.iastate.edu/news/2012/apr/chewing
**The National Science Foundation**, Estimate of Thoughts per day. http://www.nsf.gov/

# About Maggie Wilde

**Maggie is *'The Potentialist'***

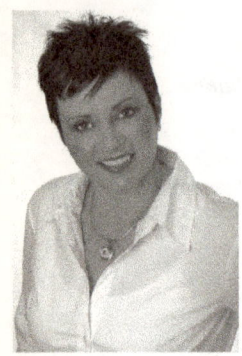

She is an inspiration to her 1000's of clients, students and audience members around the world.

Maggie's stage and education career began at 17 when she was discovered by a travelling Theatre in Education Team and *'ran away to join the circus'*. This special troupe took theatre into schools to educate and inspire. Later she began studying Psychology in the UK which sparked her passion for training in the field of Hypnosis and aligned modalities. Over the years she has used these skills to manage and overcome multiple health challenges such as systemic organ damage including kidney failure, skin, heart and lung issues, weight issues and depression. After a stroke and multiple brain seizures in 2005, those close to her were given a grim prognosis.

Maggie's passion for understanding the power of the mind had now become her life calling for a very personal reason. She drew upon her skills to recuperate and is now a walking testament to the potential within us all.

Maggie has written numerous books and authored a variety of audio programs, workshops and courses. Individual titles in the **Mind Potential Series** covering a variety of issues, each come with a tailored version of her CPR *Mind Potential Kit including unique CPR strategies and audios™* to support each title. Topics covered include: heal your body, conquering habits, emotional healing, wealth creation and building healthy relationships. She provides one on one therapy, mentoring and group workshops, seminars and webinars around the world.

www.thepotentialist.com www.maggiewilde.com
**Facebook:** www.facebook.com/maggiewildeauthor
**Twitter:** www.twitter.com/maggiewilde    **LinkedIn:** www.linkedin.in.maggiewilde

# About Sharny & Julius Kieser

## Sharny Kieser

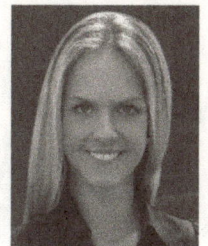

Renegade fitness experts Sharny and Julius Kieser shot to stardom when their first book, *Never Diet Again* was released in June 2011. The book was an adaptation of a step by step 'escape the diet trap' program that they had created for their private clients. They are regulars on daytime TV, radio and newspapers in their home country of Australia.

## Julius Kieser

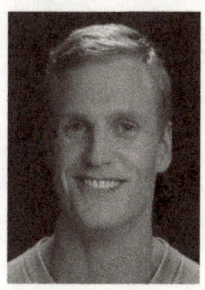

Their second book *FITlosophy 1* is "a collection of parables for athletes". It is a profound set of philosophical viewpoints that cut right to the heart of the human condition. Brutally honest, courageous, confronting, and often humorous, the stories told in this book reveal a part of the human psyche readers didn't even know was there. This book will sit with the reader for a long time after the words have actually been read.

They have also written a children's book *Where Have all The Pixies Gone?*

The couple have four children and plan on having one more. Sharny is the high-energy super mum personality in the couple. Julius' often deep, philosophical nature is contrasted by his wicked sense of humour.

www.sharnyandjulius.com          www.neverdietagainbook.com
www.neverdietagain.tv            www.yummymummy.tv

265

# Stuart Walter

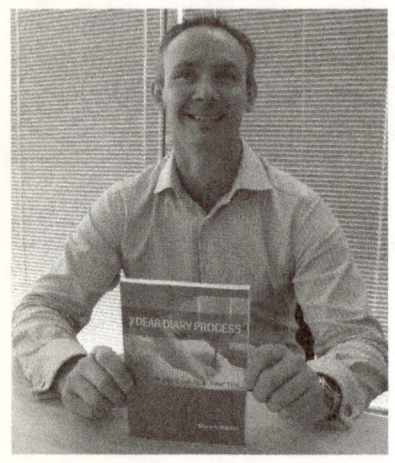

Stuart Walter, the Creator and Author, is known as the Athlete's Secret Weapon and is based in Brisbane, Australia.

It was while working with one of his professional golfers that a comment was made. That comment was the catalyst for this process, as they were sitting and talking the idea kept evolving. Results created the opportunity for this to be published, initially as a tool for all his Sporting and Business champions, now this published book is spreading around the world.

The amazing process is transforming lives...overnight. When you use *The Dear Diary Process* you can create tomorrow's outcomes today.

Deceptively simple, *The Dear Diary Process* produces powerful results. The book outlines Stuart's process and offers guidance and encouragement. It provides space for months of diary entries. www.athletessecretweapon.com

*"I've used The Dear Diary Process myself and seen progress in my goals from day 1. I recommend it to clients to help them move toward their desired outcomes."*

**Maggie Wilde**
The Potentialist, Author & Therapist

**Feel Slim and Healthy...**

**In your mind, heart, spirit and body...**

**With love from**

Maggie Wilde

◆

Email me if you wish to share your experience of the strategies in the book and the CPR audios. If you have questions or require guidance or encouragement, drop me a line too. Please be aware it might take me a few days to get back to you, but I will get back to you ... let's do this together!

Wherever you are in the world, we can connect. I offer online one on one support and mentorship via Skype and email. I provide regular workshop and seminar tours. We can even connect through live webinars and online get togethers.

You're not alone! Let's make Slim & Healthy Easy!

info@thepotentialist.com

www.thepotentialist.com